James Weir

The psychical Correlation of religious Emotion and sexual Desire

James Weir

The psychical Correlation of religious Emotion and sexual Desire

ISBN/EAN: 9783337130916

Printed in Europe, USA, Canada, Australia, Japan

Cover: Foto ©ninafisch / pixelio.de

More available books at **www.hansebooks.com**

The Psychical Correlation
of Religious Emotion
and Sexual Desire.

BY

JAMES WEIR, Jr., M. D.

SECOND EDITION.

LOUISVILLE, KY.:
COURIER-JOURNAL JOB PRINTING CO.
1897.

PREFACE TO FIRST EDITION.

The author of this monograph has been incited to its publication by the commendations of three of the most eminent critics and editors of magazines in the United States, to whom it was submitted in manuscript. In this essay, he discusses his subject from a physio-psychical standpoint, and believes that he has kept intact the canons of scientific investigation, observation, and discussion.

"Waveland," June 8, 1897.

PREFACE TO SECOND EDITION.

In preparing *The Psychical Correlation of Religious Emotion and Sexual Desire* for its second edition, the author has incorporated in it a considerable amount of additional evidence in support of his theory. He has carefully verified all references; he has endeavored to eliminate all unnecessary material; and, finally, he has changed the style of the work by dividing it into three parts, thus greatly simplifying the text. He feels under many obligations to his critics, both to those who thought his little book worthy of commendation, and to those who deemed his premises and conclusions erroneous. He feels grateful to the former, because they have caused him to believe that he has added somewhat to the literature of science; he thanks the latter, because in pointing out that which they considered untrue, they have forced him to a new and more searching study of the questions involved, thereby strengthening his belief in the truthfulness of his conclusions.

To the second edition of *The Psychical Correlation of Religious Emotion and Sexual Desire*, the author has seen fit to add certain other essays. In preparing these essays for publication, he has borrowed freely from his published papers, therefore, he desires to thank the publishers of the *New York Medical Record*, *Century Magazine*, *Denver*

Medical Times, Charlotte Monthly and *American Naturalist* for granting him permission to use such of his published material (belonging to them) as he saw fit.

The author asks the indulgence of the reader for certain repetitions in the text. These have not been occasioned by any lack of data, but occur simply because he believes that an argument is rendered stronger and more convincing by the frequent use of the same data whenever and wherever it is possible to use them. When this plan is followed, the reader, so the author believes, becomes familiar with the author's line of thought, and is, consequently, better able to comprehend and appreciate his meaning.

Finally, the author has been led to the publication of these essays by a firm belief in the truthfulness of the propositions advanced therein. He may not live to see these propositions accepted, yet he believes that, in the future, perhaps, in worthier and more able hands, they will be so weightily and forcibly elaborated and advanced that their verity will be universally acknowledged.

"Waveland," September 17, 1897.

CONTENTS.

THE PSYCHICAL CORRELATION OF RELIGIOUS EMOTION AND SEXUAL DESIRE.

PSYCHICAL PROBLEMS.

PART I.

The Origin of Religious Feeling.

I believe that man originated his first ideas of the supernatural from the external phenomena of nature which were perceptible to one or more of his five senses; his first theogony was a natural one and one taken directly from nature. Spencer, on the contrary, maintains that in man, "the first traceable conception of a supernatural being is the conception of a ghost."[1]

Primitive man's struggle for existence was so very severe that his limited sagacity was fully occupied in obtaining food and shelter; many thousands of years must have passed away before he evolved any idea of weapons other than stones and clubs. When he arrived at a psychical acuteness that originated traps, spears, bows and arrows, his struggle for ex-

---

(1) Spencer, *Principles of Sociology*, vol. 1, p. 281.

istence became easier and he had leisure to
notice the various natural phenomena by
which he was surrounded. Man evolved a
belief in a god long before he arrived at a
conception of a ghost, double, or soul. He
soon discovered that his welfare was mainly
dependent on nature, consequently he began
to propitiate nature, and finally ended by
creating a system of theogony founded on
nature alone.

"It is an evident historical fact that man
first personified natural phenomena, and then
made use of these personifications to personify
his own inward acts, his psychical ideas and
conceptions. This was the necessary process,
and external idols were formed before those
which were internal and peculiar to himself." [2]
Sun, moon, and star; mountain, hill, and dale;
torrent, waterfall, and rill, all became to him
distinct personalities, powerful beings, that
might do him great harm or much good. He
therefore endeavored to propitiate them, just

---

(2) Tito Vignoli, *Myth and Science*, p. 85.

as a dog endeavors to get the good will of
man by abjectly crawling toward him on his
belly and licking his feet. There was no element of true worship in the propitiatory
offerings of primitive man; in the beginning
he was essentially a materialist—he became a
spiritualist later on. Man's first religion must
have been, necessarily, a material one; he
worshiped (propitiated) only that which he
could see, or feel, or hear, or touch; his undeveloped psychical being could grasp nothing
higher; his limited understanding could not
frame an idea involving a spiritual element
such as animism undoubtedly presents. Ap-
ropos of the dream birth of the soul, all ter-
restrial mammals dream, and in some of them,
notably the dog and monkey, an observer can
almost predicate the subject of their dreams
by watching their actions while they are under dream influence; yet no animal save man,
as far as we know, has ever evolved any idea
of ghost or soul. It may be said, on the other
hand, that since animals show, unmistakably,

that they are, in a measure, fully conscious of
certain phenomena in the economy of nature,
and while I am not prepared to state that
any element of worship enters into their regard, I yet believe that an infinitesimal increase in the development of their psychical
beings would, undoubtedly, lead some of
them to a natural religion such as our pithecoid ancestors practiced.

The Egyptians noticed, over four thousand
years ago, that cynocephali, the dog-headed
apes of the Nile Valley, were in the habit of
welcoming the rising sun with dancing and
with howls of joy! "The habit of certain
monkeys (cynocephali) assembling, as it were,
in full court, and chattering noisily at sunrise
and sunset, would almost justify the, as yet,
uncivilized Egyptians in intrusting them with
the charge of hailing the god morning and
evening as he appeared in the east or passed
away in the west." [3]   An English fox-terrier

_____

(3) Maspero (Sayce): *The Dawn of Civilization*, p. 103, and
Maspero: *Etudes de Mythologie et d'Archiologie Egyptiennes*,
vol. ii, pp. 34, 35.

of my acquaintance is very much afraid of
thunder or any noise simulating thunder. A
load of coal rushing through a chute into the
coal cellar will send him, trembling and
alarmed, to his hiding-place beneath a bed.
This dog has never been shot over, nor has
he, as far as I know, ever heard the sound of
a gun. I am confident that he considers the
thunder as being supernatural, and that he
would propitiate it, if he only knew how.

It is not probable that, at the present time,
there exists a race of people which has not
formulated an idea of ghosts or soul; yet in
ancient times, and up to a century or so ago,
there existed many peoples who had not conceived any idea of ghosts or doubles.

According to Maspero, Sayce, Champollion,
and other Egyptologists, the ancient Egyptians probably had a natural theogony long
before they arrived at any idea of a double.
In the beginning they treated the double or
ghost with scant ceremony; it was only after
many years that an element of worship entered

into their treatment of the ghosts of their dead ancestors. They believed, at first, that the double dwelt forever in the tomb along with the dead body; afterward, they evolved the idea that the double of the dead man journeyed to the "Islands of the Blessed," where it was judged by Osiris according to its merits.[4] We have no reason for believing that the ancient Hebrews at the time of the Exodus had any knowledge of, or belief in, the existence of the soul or double, yet, that they did believe in the supernatural can not be questioned.* When Cook touched at Tierra del Fuego, he found a people in whom there existed mental habitudes but little above those to be found in the anthropoid apes. They had no knowledge whatever of the soul or double and but a dim concept of the powers of nature; they had not yet advanced far

---

(4) Maspero (Sayce): *The Dawn of Civilization*, p. 183 *et seq.*

* That the patriarchs had their household gods, we have every reason for believing; these household gods were, however, tutelary divinities, such as were kept in the house of every Chaldean, and were not the images of ancestors. Rachael, the wife of Jacob, stole the household gods of Laban, her father, who is called a Syrian. Abraham himself was a Chaldean. Gen. 11:31; also Gen. 31:19-20.

enough in psychical development to evolve any consistent form of natural theogony. They had only a shadowy concept of evil beings, powers of the air that inhabited the dense brakes of the forest, whom it would be dangerous to molest. Father Junipero Serra declares that when he first established the Mission Dolores, the Ahwashtees, Ohlones, Romanos, Altahmos, Tuolomos, and other Californian tribes had no word in their language for god, ghost, or devil.[5] The Inca Yupangui informed Balboa that there were many tribes in the interior which had no idea of ghost or soul.[6] Another writer says, that the Chirihuanas did not worship anything either in heaven or on earth, and that they had no belief whatever in a future state.[7] Modern travelers have, however, found distinct evidences of phallic worship in certain observances and customs of this tribe.[8]

(5) Bancroft: *The Native Races of the Pacific States of North America*, vol. 1, p. 400.

(6) Balboa: *History of Peru.*

(7) Garcilasso: *The Royal Commentaries of the Incas*

(8) Browlow: *Travels*, p. 136.

2

Certain autochthons of India, when first discovered, were exceedingly immature in religious beliefs; they had neither god nor devil;
they wandered through the woods subsisting
on berries and fruits, and such small animals
as their undeveloped and feeble sagacity allowed them to capture and slay. They did
not even provide themselves with shelter, but,
in pristine nakedness, roamed the forests of
the Ghauts, animals but slightly above the
anthropoid apes in point of intelligence. "In
Central California we find," says Bancroft,
"whole tribes subsisting on roots, herbs, and
insects; having no boats, no clothing, no laws,
no God."[9]

In the northwestern corner of the American continent there dwells a primitive race,
which, for the sake of unification, I will style
the Aleutians. When these people were first
discovered they were in that state of social
economics which they had reached after thousands of years of psychical and social evolu-

(9) Bancroft: *The Native Races of the Pacific States of North America*, vol. 1, p. 400.

tiou; a primitive people, such as our own ancestors were iu the very beginning of civilization. The word civilization is used advisedly; civilization is comparative, aud its degrees begin with the inception of man himself.

In their theogony, the Aleutians had arrived at an idea of the double or soul, thus showing that their religion had progressed several steps toward abstraction, that triumph of civilized religiosity; yet there remained enough veneration of natural objects to show that the origin of the religious feeling began, with them, in nature-propitiation. The bladder of the bear, which viscus, iu the estimation of the Aleutians, is the seat of life, is at once suspended above the entrance of the *kachim* and worshiped by the hunter who has slain the beast from which it was taken. Moreover, when the bear falls beneath the weapons of an Aleutian, the man begs pardon of the beast and prays the latter to forgive him and to do him no harm. "A hunter who has struck a

mortal blow generally remains within his hut
for one or several days, according to the importance of the slain animal."[10] The first
herring that is caught is showered with compliments and blessings; pompous titles are
lavished upon it, and it is handled with the
greatest respect and reverence; it is the her-
ring-god![11]

Sidné, chief god of the Aleutian theogony,
on final analysis, is found to be the Earth,
mother of all things. The *angakouts*, or priests,
of this people individualize and deify, however, all the phenomena of nature; there are
cloud-gods, sea-gods, river-gods, fire-gods,
rain-gods, storm-gods, etc., etc., etc. Everywhere, throughout all nature, the Inoit, or
Aleutian system of theology, penetrates,
stripped, it is true, of much of its original
materialism, yet retaining enough to show its
undoubted origin in the sensual percepts, recepts, and concepts of its primal founders.

---

(10) Reclus: *Primitive Folk*, p. 18.
(11) Dall: *Alaska and its Resources*, p. 96.

As I have observed above, the religion of these people has gained a certain degree of abstraction, and this abstraction is further shown by the presence of certain phallic rites and ceremonies in their religious observances; but of this, more anon.

In most of the tribes of Equatorial Africa, nature-worship has been superseded by ghost-worship, devil-worship, or witch-worship, or, rather, by ghost, devil, or witch propitiation; yet, in the sanctity of the fetich, which is everywhere present, we see a relic of nature-worship. Moreover, many of these tribes deify natural phenomena, such as the sun, the moon, the stars, thunder, lightning, etc., etc., etc., showing that here, too, in all probability, religious feeling had its origin in nature propitiation.

Abstraction also enters, to a certain extent, into the religious beliefs of most of these negroes, in whom primal materialism has given place to the unbridled superstition of crude spiritism. The curious habit these

people have of scraping a little bone dust
from the skull of a dead ancestor and then
eating it with their food, thus, as they think,
transmitting from the dead to the living the
qualities of the former, is close kin to, and, in
my opinion, is probably derived from, a worship of the generative principle.   When we
take into consideration the fact that circumcision, *extensio clitoridis*, and other phallic rites
are exceedingly common and prevalent among
these negroes, this opinion has strong evidence in its support.[12]

The Wa-kamba may have some idea of immortality, though observers have never been
able to determine this definitely.   " The dead
bodies of chiefs are not thrown to the hyenas,
as with the Masai, but are carefully buried
instead. . . . The bodies of less important
members of the tribe are simply thrown to
the hyenas." [13]

(12) Negroes of Benin and Sierra Leone (Bosman, *loc. cit.*, p.
528), Mandingoes (Waitz, vol. ii, p. 3), Bechuanas (Holub,
loc. cit., p. 398); quoted also by Westermarck, *Human Marriage*,
p. 206
(13) Gregory : *The Great Rift Valley*, p. 351.

In this people, religious ideas are exceedingly primitive and indefinite. They seem to
propitiate nature, however, when they wish
rain, for they offer up to the rain-spirit votive
offerings of bananas, grain, and beer, which
they place beneath the trees. This seems to be
their only religious rite according to Gregory,
who, in all probability is in error. For, in
the next sentence, he informs us that these
negroes practice circumcision. He thinks
that they perform this operation for sanitary
reasons, "as the natives have continually to
ford streams and wade through swamps
abounding in the larvæ of *Bilharzia hæmaturia*,
the rite no doubt lessens the danger of incur-
ring hæmaturia." [14] This is bestowing upon
ignorant and savage negroes a psychical acuteness which far transcends that of the laity of
civilized races! What do the Wa-kamba
know of sanitation, hæmaturia, and the larva
of Bilharzia! Circumcision among these people always occurs at puberty, and is, unques-

---

(14) Gregory: *The Great Rift Valley*, p. 351.

tionably, a phallic rite. Parenthetically, it
may be stated here that a few of the primitive peoples still in existence appear to have
grasped the idea of the life-giving principle,
and to have established worship of the *func-
tio generationis* without having experienced
certain preliminary psychical stages necessary
for its evolution from nature-worship. I believe, however, that this is apparent and not
real; nature-worship, very probably, at one
time existed among all these people.

The Kikuyu have a very elaborate system
of theogony, in which all of the phenomena
of nature with which they are acquainted are
deified. A goat is invariably sacrificed to the
sun when they set out on a journey, and its
blood is carried along and sprinkled on the
paths and bridges in order to appease the
spirits of the forest and the river.

Stuhlmann places this tribe among the
Bantu; from the evidence of other observers,
however, they seem to be Nilotic Hamites, and

belong properly to the Masai. [15] This would
account for the similarity of method in circumcision, which, among both Kikuyu and
Masai, is incomplete. Johnston calls attention to this very peculiar method and describes it minutely in a Latin foot-note. [16]

The Masai are mixed devil, nature, and
phallic worshipers; the last mentioned cult
being evolved, beyond question, from nature-
worship. It may be set down as an established fact that, where nature-worship does
not exist in some form or other among primitive peoples, phallic worship is likewise absent.
Indeed, such peoples generally have no religious feeling whatever. They may have some
shadowy idea of an evil spirit like the "*Auri-
mwantya dsongo ngombe auri kinemu,*" the
Old Man of the Woods [17] of the Wa-poko-
mo, but that is all.

Carl Lumholtz, writing of the Australians,
says: "The Australian blacks do not, like

(15) Stuhlmann: *Mit Emin Pasha*, p. 848.
(16) Johnston: *The Kilima-Njaro Expedition*, p. 412.
(17) Gregory: *The Great Rift Valley*, p. 344.

many other savage tribes, attach any ideas of
divinity to the sun or moon. On one of our
expeditions the full moon rose large and red
over the palm forest. Struck by the splendor of the scene, I pointed at the moon and
asked my companions, 'Who made it?'
They answered 'Other blacks.' Thereupon
I asked, 'Who made the sun?' and got the
same answer. The natives also believe that
they themselves can produce rain, particularly
with the help of wizards. To produce rain
they call *milka*. When on our expeditions
we were overtaken by violent tropical storms,
my blacks always became enraged at the
strangers who had caused the rain." [18] In
regard to their belief in the existence of a
double or soul, the same author sums up as
follows : " Upon the whole, it may be said
that these children of nature are unable to
conceive a human soul independent of the
body, and the future life of the individual lasts
no longer than his physical remains." [19] Mr.

---

(18) Lumholtz: *Among Cannibals*, p. 282.
(19) *Ibid.*, p. 270.

Mann, of New South Wales, who, according to Lumholtz, has made a thirty years' study of the Australians, says that the natives have no religion whatever, except fear of the "devil-devil." [20] Another writer, and one abundantly qualified to judge, says that they acknowledge no supreme being, have no idols, and believe only in an evil spirit whom they do not worship. They say that this spirit is afraid of fire, so they never venture abroad after dusk without a fire-stick. [21]

"I verily believe we have arrived at the sum total of their religion, if a superstitious dread of the unknown can be so designated. Their mental capacity does not admit of their grasping the higher truths of pure religion," says Eden. [22]

In these savages we see a race whose psychical status is so low in the intellectual scale that they have not evolved any idea of the

(20) Lumholtz: *Among Cannibals*, p. 283.

(21) *Ibid.*, p. 283.

(22) Eden: *The Fifth Continent*, p. 69; quoted also by Lumholtz: *Among Cannibals*.

double or soul. The mental capacity of the Australians, I take it, is no lower than was that of any race (no matter how intellectual it may be at the present time) at one period of its history. All races have a tendency toward psychical development under favorable surroundings; it has been a progress instead of a decadence, a rise instead of a fall!

There are yet other people who believe in the supernatural, yet who have no idea of immortality. When Gregory ascended the glacier of Mount Kenya, the water froze in the cooking-pots which had been filled overnight. His carriers were terribly alarmed by the phenomenon, and swore that the water was bewitched! The explorer scolded them for their silliness and bade them set the pots on the fire, which, having been done, "the men sat round and anxiously watched; when it melted they joyfully told me that the demon was expelled, and I told them they could now use the water; but as soon as my back was turned they poured it away, and refilled their pots from an adjoining brook." [23]

Stanley declares that no traces of religious feeling can be found in the Wahuma. "They believe most thoroughly in the existence of an evil influence in the form of a man, who exists in uninhabited places, as a wooded, darksome gorge, or large extent of reedy brake, but that he can be propitiated by gifts; therefore the lucky hunter leaves a portion of the meat, which he tosses, however, as he would to a dog, or he places an egg, or a small banana, or a kid-skin, at the door of the miniature dwelling, which is always at the entrance to the zeriba." [24]

This observer shows that he does not know the true meaning of the word religion; the example that he gives demonstrates the fact that these negroes *do* have religious feeling. The simple act of offering propitiatory gifts to the "evil influence" is, from the very nature

(23) Gregory: *The Great Rift Valley*, p. 170,
(24) Stanley: *In Darkest Africa*, vol. 11, p. 400.

of the deed, a religious observance. Further-
more, these savages have charms and fetiches
innumerable, which, in my opinion, are relics
of nature-worship. The miniature house
mentioned by Stanley is common to the majority of the equatorial tribes, and seems to
be a kind of common fetich ; *i. e.*, one that is
enjoyed by the entire tribe. It is mentioned
by Du Chaillu, Chaillé Long, Stanley, and
many others. [25]

Du Chaillu tells of one tribe, the Bakalai,
in which the women worship a particular
divinity named Njambai. [26] This writer is
even more inexact than Stanley, hence, we
get very little scientific data from his volumi-
nous works. From what he says of Njambai,
I am inclined to believe that he is a negro
Priapus ; this, however, is a conjectural belief and has no scientific warrant.

The Tucúna Indians of the Amazon Valley,
who resemble the Passés, Jurís, and Muahés

---

(25) Du Chaillu: *Equatorial Africa;* Chaillé Long : *Naked
Truths of Naked People;* Stanley : *In Darkest Africa.*
(26) Du Chaillu: *Equatorial Africa,* p. 240.

in physical appearance and customs, social and otherwise, are devil-worshipers. They are very much afraid of the *Jupari*, or devil, who seems to be " simply a mischievous imp, who is at the bottom of all those mishaps of their daily life, the causes of which are not very immediate or obvious to their dull understandings. The idea of a Creator or a beneficent God has not entered the minds of these Indians." [27]

The Peruvians, at the time of the Spanish conquest, worshiped nature; that is, the sun was deified under the name of *Pachacamac*, the Giver of Life, and was worshiped as such. The Inca, who was his earthly representative, was likewise his chief priest, though there was a great High Priest, or *Villac Vmu*, who stood at the head of the hierarchy, but who was second in dignity to the Inca. [28] The moon, wife of the sun, the stars, thunder, lightning, and other natural phenomena were also deified. But, as it invariably happens, where nature-

(27) Bates : *The Naturalist on the River Amazon*, p. 381.
(28) Prescott : *The Conquest of Peru*, vol. 1, p. 101.

worship is allowed to undergo its natural evolution, certain elements of phallic worship had
made their appearance. These I will discuss
later on.

The great temple of the sun was at Cuzco,
"where, under the munificence of successive
sovereigns, it had become so rich that it received the name of Coricancha, or 'the Place
of Gold.'" [29] According to the *relacion* of
Sarmiento, and the commentaries of Garcilasso and other Spanish writers, this building,
which was surrounded by chapels and smaller
edifices, and which stood in the heart of the
city, must have been truly magnificent with
its lavish adornments of virgin gold!

Unlike the Aztecs, a kindred race of people,
the Peruvians rarely sacrificed human beings
to their divinities, but, like the religion of the
former, the religion of the latter had become
greatly developed along ceremonial lines, as
we will see later on in this essay.

It is a far cry from Peru to Japan, from the

---

(29) Prescott: *The Conquest of Peru*, vol. 1, p. 95.

Incas to the Ainus, yet these widely separated
races practiced religions that were almost
identical in point of fundamental principles.
Both worshiped nature, but the Peruvians
were far ahead of the Ainus in civilization,
and their religion, as far as ritual and ceremony are concerned, far surpassed that of the
" Hairy Men" when viewed from an æsthetic
standpoint. Ethically, I am inclined to
believe the religion of the Ainus is just as
high as was that of the Incas.

Literature is indebted to the Rev. John
Batchelor for that which is, probably, the
most readable book that has ever been published about these interesting people; from a
scientific standpoint, however, this work is
greatly lacking. Many ethnologists and
anthropologists considered the Ainu autoch-
thonic to Japan; I am forced to conclude
from the evidence, however, that he is an
emigrant, and that he came originally from
North China or East Siberia. Be he emigrant
or indigene, one thing is certain, namely, that

3

he has been an inhabitant of the Japanese Archipelago for thousands of years. The oldest book in the Japanese language has this in it anent the Ainus: "When our august ancestors descended from heaven in a boat, they found upon this island several barbarous races, the most fierce of whom were the Ainu." [29]

The Ainu is probably the purest type of primitive man in existence. I had been led to believe by the work of Miss Bird [30] that these people were on a par with the Australians, and that they had no religious ideas whatever. (Vogt seems to advance this conclusion also, [31] while De Quatrefages [32*] appears to have omitted this people from his tabulation. Peschel places them among the Giliaks on the Lower Amoor, and the inhabitants of the Kurile Islands. [33] These tribes

(29) Batchelor: *The Ainu of Japan*, p. 13.

(30) Bird: *Unbeaten Tracks in Japan.*

(31) Vogt: *Lectures on Man.*

(32) De Quatrefages: *The Human Species.*

(*) De Quatrefages, in his *Hommes Fossiles*, places the Ainus anthropologically among the Primeval Teutons!

(33) Peschel: *The Races of Man*, p. 388.

are mixed nature, devil, and phallic worshipers.) Batchelor, however, shows very clearly that these people *do* have a religion, and that this religion is highly developed.

Their chief god, or rather goddess (for the Ainus regard the female as being higher than the male as far as gods are concerned), is the sun.[34] Like the Peruvians, they regard the sun as the Creator, but they are unlike them in the fact. that they think that they can not reach the goddess by direct appeal. She must be addressed through intermediaries or messengers. These messengers, the goddess of the fire, the goddess of the water, etc., are in turn addressed through the agency of *inao*, or prayer-sticks. This intermediary idea is curiously like some practices of the Roman Catholic church, or, rather, of communicants, who get the saints to carry their petitions to God.

The Inao are peculiar, inasmuch as nothing exactly like them is known. The feather prayer-plumes of some of the Western Indians

(34) Batchelor: *The Ainu of Japan*, p. 89.

are used for like purposes, but these are offered directly to the Great Spirit, and not to inter-mediaries. " Inao, briefly described, are pieces of whittled willow wood, having the shavings attached to the top."[35]　Like the Aleutians, when these people kill a bear or other wild animal, they propitiate its spirit by bestowing upon it the most fulsome compliments, and, like the religion of these Indians, the religion of the Ainus has developed along natural lines, and shows certain phallic elements.

We see from the examples here given, that religious feeling had its origin in the idea of propitiation; in fact, that it was born in fear, and by fear was it fostered.　We see, further-more, that man was not created with religious feeling as a psychical trait, but that he ac-quired it later on.　We see, finally, that re-ligious feeling is based, primarily and funda-mentally, on one of the chief laws of nature —self-protection.

It is not at all probable that man in the

(35) Batchelor: *The Ainu of Japan*, p. 87.

beginning, just after his evolution from his
ape-like ancestor, had, at first, any belief whatever in supernatural agencies. In his struggle
for existence, all of his powers were directed
toward the procurement of his food and the
preservation of life; the pithecoid man was
only a degree higher than the beasts in the
scale of animal life. His psychic being, as
yet, remained, as it were, *in ovo*, and a long
period of time must have elapsed before he
began to formulate and to recognize a system
of theogony. After years of experience, during which the laws of heredity and progressive evolution played prominent parts, he took
precedence over other animals, and his struggle
for existence became easier. He then had
time to study the wonderful and, to him,
mysterious phenomena of nature. His limited
knowledge could not explain the various natural operations by which he was surrounded,
therefore he looked upon them as being mysterious and supernatural. His psychical being
became active and inquiring, to satisfy which

he created a system of gods which was founded
on natural phenomena. At first, the gods of
primitive man were, probably, few in number, and the chief god of all was the sun. Man
early recognized the sun's importance in the
economy of nature; this beautiful star, rising
in the east in the morning, marching through
the heavens during the day, and sinking behind the western horizon in the evening, must
have been, to the awakening soul of man, a
source of endless conjecture and debate. What
was more natural than his making the sun the
greatest god in his system of theogony? Man
recognized in him the source of all life, and,
when he arrived at an age when he could use
abstract ideation in formulating his religion,
he deified the life-giving function as he
noticed it in himself; he began to worship the
generative principle. Solar worship and its
direct descendant, phallic worship, at one
time or another were the religions of almost
every race on the face of the globe. Solar
worship, owing to its material quality, has

long since been abandoned by civilized man ; but phallic worship, the first *abstract* religion evolved by man, has taken deeper root; its fundamental principles are still present, though they have their seat in our subliminal consciousness, and we are, therefore, not actively conscious of their existence. But before entering on the discussion of this last point, let us turn for a time to a study of phallic worship.

PART II.

Phallic Worship.

Phallic worship, in some form or other, has been practiced by almost every race under the sun. Indeed, among primitive peoples, those who do not practice this cult are so few in number that they have, practically, no weight whatever in a discussion of this subject. Moreover, those primitive peoples who do not worship the generative principle, either directly or indirectly, are without any religion whatsoever, and are the very lowest of all mankind in point of intelligence. I have only to cite the Tierra del Fuegians, the Bushmen, the Australians, and the Akka or Ticki-Ticki, the Pygmies of Central Africa, to prove the truthfulness of this assertion.

D'Hancarville, in his magnificent work, has traced the progress of the worship of the generative principle over the entire world, while Knight, in his scholarly essay,[36] has brought out its psychological truths in a manner which can not be surpassed. It is not my purpose to enter into a detailed account of this cult; I propose rather to discuss its probable origin in the beginning, and to give a brief outline of its history, as it is to be observed among living peoples. I wish to show, also, its connection with certain religious ceremonies and festivals of Christian peoples,which had their origin, *ab initio*, in the worship of Priapus. And, before beginning the discussion of this subject, I beg to remind the reader that a priest of Priapus regarded his sistrum as being just as sacred as a Catholic priest now considers any vessel or robe used in the service of mass, and that the priests of Brahma look on the Lingam with as much reverence and awe as did the Levites on the Ark of the Covenant and the Holy of Holies. Phallic worship is a religion, the oldest *abstract* religion in existence. Funda-

---

(36) Knight: *The Worship of Priapus.*

mentally the Creator — the Life Giver — is the
phallic worshiper's god.   Is he very far wrong
in all that is absolutely essential?   " Men think
they know because they are sure they feel,
and are firmly convinced because strongly
agitated.   Hence proceed that haste and vio-
lence with which devout persons of all religious condemn the rites and doctrines of
others, and the furious zeal and bigotry with
which they maintain their own, while, perhaps, if both were equally understood, both
would be found to have the same meaning,
and only to differ in the modes of conveying
it." [37]

The Pueblo Indians of New Mexico are
worshipers of the generative principle, and,
like most religious sects, have evolved some
very curious rites and ceremonies.   The
ancient temple of Venus or Aphrodite were
filled with *hetæræ*, who were necessary adjuncts for the proper performance of the mysteries of Priapus.   These Indians, however,

æ

---

(37) Knight: *The Worship of Priapus*, p. 14.

will not allow women to enter into their
sacred ceremonies, but, on the contrary, emas-
culate men (by occasioning organic and func-
tional degeneration of the sexual organs), who
serve as hetaræ to the chiefs and shamans or
priests. These androgynes are called *mujerados*, a term which describes their sexual condition.

"In order to cultivate a mujerado, a very
powerful man is chosen, and he is made to
masturbate excessively and ride constantly.
Gradually such irritable weakness of the
genital organs is engendered that, in riding,
great loss of semen is induced. This condition of irritability passes into paralytic impotence. Then the testicles and penis atrophy,
the hair of the beard falls out, the voice loses
its depth and compass, and physical strength
and energy decrease. Inclinations and dis-
position become feminine. The mujerado
loses his position in society as a man. He
takes on feminine manners and customs, and
associates with women; yet, for religious rea-

sons, he is held in high honor." [38] The phallic
ceremonies of the Pueblos take place in the
spring, when the life principle is exceedingly
active throughout all nature.

In all probability the " botes" of the Mon-
tana Indians and the "burdachs" of the
Washington tribes serve as masculine hetæræ
to the chiefs and medicine men, though this
has not been definitely determined.   Dr.
Holder described a typical "bote" of the
Absaroke tribe in the New York Medical
Journal, 1889.   This androgyne, in many respects, resembled the mujerados of the Pueblo
Indians, and probably served a like purpose
in his tribe.

According   to Ross, a   Konyaga woman,
when she has a good-looking boy, dresses him
in girl's clothes and brings him up as a female.
When he arrives at a suitable age he is sent
to wait on the priests of the tribe and is introduced by them into the sacred mysteries of

(38) Krafft-Ebing: *Psychopathia Sexualis*, p. 201; see also
Hammond: *Impotence in the Male.*

their cult; in fact, he becomes a masculine hetæra.

When we read of such things we feel pretty much as Herodotus felt when he saw the naked women of Mendes submitting themselves openly (ες επιδειξιν ανθρωπων) to the embraces of the sacred goat.* To the Greek historian this act was simply horrible (τερας); and yet these Egyptians experienced no repugnance whatever. To them it represented the incarnation of the deity, and was, therefore, a sacred and holy action, just as masculine hetarism is regarded as a holy profession among the Konyagas. Phallic hetarism is one of the sacraments of the Konyaga church, and, as such, it is held in all that reverence and awe with which the savage devotee endows the mysteries of his faith.†

(*) Herodotus: *Euterpe*, 46.

(†) Masculine hetarism is still in vogue among many primitive peoples, and is distinctly a religious rite. "The Kanats of New Caledonia frequently assemble at night in a cabin to give themselves up to this kind of debauchery. . . . In the whole of America, from north to south, similar customs have existed or still exist." Letourneau: *The Evolution of Marriage*, p. 62. The same author says: "It

The ancient Hebrews, ancestors of one of the most ancient of the civilized races of the earth, held it in high honor. Even wise King Solomon, in the days of his old age, turned from the abstractly pure religion of his father " to Astoreth, the goddess of the Zidonians, and to Milcom, the abomination of the Ammonites." [39] He was guilty of constructing a " high place " for Chemosh, " the abomination of Moab." [40] Any good modern biblical encyclopedia will tell the reader about Astoreth and her worship, and what the " high places " and the " groves " were.

Even the " good kings," such as Asa, Amaziah, *et al.*, did not remove the high places and

(39) *I Kings :* chap. xi, verse 5.
(40) *Ibid.,* verse 7.

---

was also a widely spread custom throughout Polynesia, and even a special deity presided over it. The Southern Californians did the same, and the Spanish missionaries, on their arrival in the country, found men dressed as women and assuming their part. They were trained to this from youth, and often publicly married to the chiefs. Nero was evidently a mere plagiarist. The existence of analogous customs has been proved against the Guyacurus of La Plata, the natives of the Isthmus of Darien, the tribes of Louisiana, and the ancient Illinois."

the groves, for we read that, notwithstanding the fact that these kings did that which was right in the sight of the Lord, they did not remove the high places. In the case of Amaziah, it is written:

" And he did that which was right in the sight of the Lord, yet not like David, his father; he did according to all things as Joash, his father, did.

" Howbeit, the high places were not taken away: as yet the people did sacrifice and burnt incense on the high places." [41] All of the so-called " wicked kings " were phallic worshipers, and both male and female hetarism flourished during their reigns. We read of Josiah, a " good king," " And he broke down the houses of the sodomites (*kedescheim*) that were by the house of the Lord." [42] Here, in unmistakable terms (*kedescheim*), the phallic act of the hetara is specified.

---

(41) *II Kings:* chap. xiv, verses 3, 4.
(42) *Ibid.*, chap. xxiii, verse 7.

Herodotus wrote: "Almost all mankind consort with women in their sacred temples, except in Greece and Egypt." [43] This is a queer mistake for a Greek to make, yet this historian is noted for his unreliability, and we should not feel surprised at this gross error. Concerning the Aphrodite of Abydos, what she was and what took place in her temples, is a matter of history. Indeed, this goddess was surnamed *Porne!* In Corinth, delubral hetarism was openly practiced; also at Bubastis and Naucratis in Egypt. Royal princesses were pallacides in the temple of Ammon; in fact, they took pride in the title of *pallakis!* * "It is known what excessive debauchery took place in the 'groves' and 'high places' of the 'Great Goddess.' The custom

---

(43) Herodotus: *Euterpe*, 64.

(*) Strabo, when writing of the Armenians, who were phallic worshipers, says: "It is the custom of the most illustrious personages to consecrate their virgin daughters to this goddess (Anaïtis). This in no way prevents them from finding husbands, even after they have prostituted themselves for a long time in the temples of Anaïtis. No man feels on this account any repugnance to take them as wives." Strabo: vol. xi, 14; quoted also by Letourneau: *The Evolution of Marriage*, p. 46.

was so deeply rooted that in the grotto of
Bethlehem what was done formerly in the
name of Adonis is done to-day in the name
of the Virgin Mary by Christian pilgrims;
and the Mussulman *hadjis* do likewise in the
sanctuaries of Mecca!" [44]

But let us return to primitive peoples,
from whose customs and beliefs we can learn
what our own ancestors must have believed
before the besom of civilization swept aside
the crudities of savagery.

The Khonds of India are phallic worshipers, and, in the practice of their religion,
Priapus saves many a girl who would be,
otherwise, offered up on the bloody altars of
their divinities. The pregnant woman is
sacred, hence, religious prostitution is exceedingly prevalent. But it frequently happens
that some unfortunate creature, who is not
pleasing to the shamans, is seized, tied to the
stake and butchered.[45] As the blood flows

---

(44) Reclus: *Primitive Folk*, p. 69; Sepp: *Heidenthum u. Christenthum.*

(45) Sherwill: *The Rajmahal Hills.*

4

down and deluges the ground, "the divine spirit enters into the priest and inspires him." [46] This sacrifice is of itself a phallic rite; the blood-offering is supposed to be exceedingly acceptable to Earth, the mother of all things. Blood is the essence of the life-giving principle; hence, the essence is returned to the great Giver, as a propitiatory offering.

In point of fact, the worship of the generative principle is everywhere prevalent in India.* In the Lingam, or holy altar of the Brahmins, we see a conjunction of the male and female sexual organs, while religious prostitution, in the shape of hetarism, crowds

---

(46) Reclus: *Primitive Folk*, p. 317.

(*) Speaking of the ceremony of priestly prelibation as it was practiced in the Kingdom of Malabar, Forbes writes as follows: "The ecclesiastic power took precedence of the civil on this particular point, and the sovereign himself passed under the yoke. Like the other women, the queen had to submit to the right of prelibation exercised by the high priest, who had a right to the first three nights, and who was paid fifty pieces of gold besides for his trouble." Forbes: *Oriental Memoirs*, vol. 1, p. 446; quoted also by Letourneau: *The Evolution of Marriage*, p. 48. De Rémusat says that, in Cambodia, the daughters of poor parents retain their virginity longer than their richer sisters simply because they have not the money with which to pay the priest for defloration!

the inner courts and corridors of almost every temple in the land with hierodules and bayaderes. The Vedas abound in references, either direct or indirect, to phallic worship. Indeed, according to some authorities, the Hindu Brahma is the same as the Greek Pan, * "who is the creative spirit of the deity transfused through matter." [47]

Hundreds of pages have been written on snake-worship, in which a wonderful amount of metaphysical lore has been expended. Mr. Herbert Spencer devotes several pages to the snake, and the reason for its appearance in the religion of primitive peoples. He ascribes to savages a psychical acuteness that I am by

(*) "The people have put the idol named *Coppal* in a neighboring house; there she is served by priests and *Devadachi*, or slaves of the gods. These are prostitute girls, whose employment is to dance and to ring little bells in cadence while singing infamous songs, either in the pagoda or in the streets when the idol is carried out in state," writes Letourneau in *The Evolution of Marriage*, quoting from *Lettres édifiantes*. *Coppal* was and is a Brahminical Venus, and her worship is wholly phallic in character. The ancient Indo-Iranians worshiped a similar deity. The worship of Coppal, both in ritual and in significance, is identical with that of the Greek Aphrodite.

(47) Brugsch, Knight, Müller, *et al.*

no means willing to allow them, inasmuch as
he makes them give a psychical causation for
their adoption of the serpent as a deity, such
as no ignorant and uncultivated savage could
have possibly evolved. I am inclined to believe that, like all great students and thinkers,
Mr. Spencer has a hobby, and that this hobby
is animism or ancestor-worship. When he
gives out, as a reason for the snake's almost
universal appearance in the religions of primitive peoples, that the latter consider it an animal which has assumed the returning ghost,
double, or soul of an ancestor,[48] I think that
he is very much in error. There are very few
primitive folk, comparatively speaking, who
believe in metempsychosis. In all probability,
when a race, like the ancient Egyptians, for
instance, had reached a high degree of civilization, they idealized many of their religious
beliefs and customs; hence, the serpent probably lost its initial and simple symbolical meaning, and stood for something higher and more

(48) Spencer: *Principles of Sociology*, vol. 1, p. 798.

cthical during the reign of the great Pharoahs,
and the Golden Age of the Greeks and Latins.
I am positive, however, that the snake's original significance was wholly phallic in character, and that its adoption as a symbol was
simple and material, as I explain elsewhere in
this essay.

I am forced to this conclusion by its presence among phallic symbols in almost every
race that practiced or practices a worship of
the generative principles. The Pueblo Indians, whom I have mentioned elsewhere in
this treatise, regard the snake symbol with
reverence; the Moqui Indians have their
sacred snake dance, in which they worship
the reptiles, handling the most vicious and
poisonous rattlesnakes with seeming impu-
nity; the Apaches hold that every rattlesnake
is an emissary of the devil; [49] " the Piutes
of Nevada have a demon deity in the form of a
serpent still supposed to exist in the waters of
Pyramid Lake; " [50] on the wall of an ancient

(49) Bancroft: *Native Races, etc.*, p. 135.
(50) *Ibid.*

Aztec ruin at Palenque there is a tablet, on
which there is a cross standing on the head of
a serpent, and surmounted by a bird. "The
cross is the symbol of the four winds; the
bird and serpent the rebus of the rain-god,
their ruler."[51]   The Quiche god, Hurakan,
was called the "Strong Serpent," and the sign
of Tlaloc, the Aztec rain-god, was a golden
snake. All of these tribes are or were worshipers of the generative principles, though,
in most of them, phallic worship has or had
lost much of its original significance.[52]   In
Yucatan and elsewhere in South and Central
America, notably among the ruins of Chichen
Itza, the serpent symbol is frequently in evidence.[53]   The Indians of the Tocantins in
Brazil, as well as the Muras, Mundurucus and
Cucamas, are mixed nature and devil worshipers;* as a sequence, certain phallic rites are
to be observed in their religious ceremonies.

(51) Bancroft (Brinton): *Native Races, etc.*, p. 135.
(52) *Ibid.*, p. 134.
(53) Stephens: *Yucatan.*
(*) Consult Frantz Keller: *The Amazon and Madeira Rivers.*

Many of the native tribes of North America perform phallic rites at puberty. James Owen Dorsey, who has made a study of the Siouan cults, writes as follows :

" Every male Dakota sixteen years old and upward is a soldier, and is formally and mysteriously enlisted into the service of the war prophet. From him he receives the implements of war, carefully constructed after models furnished from the armory of the gods, painted after a divine prescription, and charged with a missive virtue — the tonwan — of the divinities. To obtain these necessary articles the proud applicant is required for a time to abuse himself and serve him, while he goes through a series of painful and exhausting performances, which are necessary on his part to enlist favorable notice of the gods. These performances consist chiefly of vapor baths, fastings, chants, prayers, and nightly vigils. The spear and the tomahawk being prepared and consecrated, the person who is to receive them approaches the wakan man (priest), and presents a pipe to him. He asks a favor, in substance as follows : ' Pity thou me, poor and helpless, a *woman*, and confer on me the ability to perform *manly* deeds.' " [54] According- ing to Miss Fletcher, when an Oglala girl arrives at puberty, a great feast is prepared, and favored guests invited thereto. "A prominent feature in the feast is the feeding of these privileged persons and the girl in whose honor the feast is given, with choke cherries, as the choicest rarity to be had in the winter. . . . In the ceremony, a few of the cherries are taken in a spoon and held over the sacred smoke and then fed to the girl." [55] This is considered one of the most sacred of their feasts.

While discussing the phallic observances of the North American races, I will introduce the subject of tattooing, though it properly belongs elsewhere in this treatise.

At puberty, the Hudson Bay Eskimos inva-

(54) Dorsey : *Siouan Cults, An. Rep. Bur. Eth.*, 1889-90, p. 444.
(55) Fletcher : *Peabody Museum Report*, vol. iii, p. 260.

riably tattoo their boys and girls. Lucien M.
Turner writing of the latter, says :

"When a girl arrives at puberty she is
taken to a secluded locality by some old
woman versed in the art of tattooing, and
stripped of her clothing. A small quantity
of half-charred lamp wick of moss is mixed
with oil from the lamp. A needle is used to
prick the skin, and the pasty substance is
smeared over the wound. The blood mixes
with it, and in a few days a dark-bluish spot
is left. The operation continues four days.
When the girl returns to the tent it is known
that she has begun to menstruate."[56] Both
Eastern and Western Inoits celebrate puberty
with certain rites. It is rather difficult, however, to get them to say much about this matter, so I will not present the evidence, meager
as it is, which has been gleaned from the
works of various explorers. One can readily
see that much of it is conjecture, therefore of
little scientific value.

(56) Turner: *An. Rep. Bur. Eth.*, 1889-90, p. 208.

Not far from the Place of Gold, the magnificent temple in which the ancient Peruvians worshiped the Life Giver, was another great edifice, styled the "House of the Virgins of the Sun." This was the domicile of the pallacides or hetaræ of the Chief Priest, the Inca. "No one but the Inca and the Coya, or queen, might enter the consecrated precincts. . . . Woe to the unhappy maiden who was detected in an intrigue! By the stern laws of the Incas she was buried alive, her lover strangled, and the town or village to which he belonged was razed to the ground and sowed with stones as if to efface every memorial of his existence. One is astonished to find so close a resemblance between the institutions of the American Indian, the ancient Roman, and the modern Catholic. Chastity and purity of life are virtues in woman that would seem to be of equal estimation with the barbarian and with the civilized — yet the ultimate destination of the inmates of these religious houses (there were hundreds of them) was materially different. . . . Though Virgins of the Sun, they were the brides of the Inca." [57] The monarch had thousands of these hetaræ in his various palaces. When he wished to lessen the number in his seraglios, he sent some of them to their own homes, where they lived ever after respected and revered as holy beings.[58] The religion of the Peruvians had reached a high degree of development, and many of the crudities of simple phallic worship had either been entirely abandoned or so idealized that they had been lost in the mists of ritual and ceremony. For "the ritual of the Incas involved a routine of observances as complex and elaborate as ever distinguished that of any nation, whether pagan or Christian." [59]

Notwithstanding the fact that the descendants of the Incas have been under the guardianship of the priests of the Catholic church

(57) Prescott : *Conquest of Peru*, vol. 1. p. 110 *et seq*.
(58) *Ibid*., p. 112.
(59) *Idid*., p. 103.

for hundreds of years, a close, careful, pains-
taking, and accurate observer informs me
that he has repeatedly noticed unmistakable
phallic rites interwoven with their Christian
ceremonials and beliefs. The same can be
said of a kindred race and a kindred religion.
Biart, writing of the descendants of the Aztecs,
says: "In grottoes unexpectedly discovered,
I have frequently found myself in the presence of a figure of Mictlanteuctli, at the foot
of which a recent offering of food had been
placed." [60] How exceedingly basic and fundamental the worship of the generative principle must be in Psychos itself, is indicated by
these facts !

In the very beginnings of history we find
that many races of people held the worship of
the generative principle in high honor. Not
only has the knowledge of this fact come to
us through the sculptured monuments of the
Egyptians and the tablets, cylinders, etc., of
the Chaldeans, but it has also been set before

(60) Biart: *The Aztecs*, p. 139.

RELIGION AND LUST. 61

us by ancient historians. Speaking of the Chaldeans Herodotus (1,199) * says, " Every woman born in the country must enter once during her life-time the inclosure of the temple of Aphrodite, must there sit down and unite herself to a stranger. Many who are wealthy are too proud to mix with the rest, and repair thither in closed chariots, followed by a considerable train of slaves. The greater number seat themselves on the sacred pavement, with a cord twisted about their ;heads,—and there is always a crowd there, coming and going; the women being divided by ropes into long lanes, down which strangers pass to make their choice. A woman who has once taken her place here can not return home until a stranger has thrown into her lap a silver coin, and has led her away with him beyond the limits of the sacred inclosure. As he throws the money he pronounces these words: ' May the goddess Mylitta make thee happy!'

---

* Herodotus: *Clio;* See also Cary's translation of Herodotus, page 86 *et seq.*

Now among the Assyrians, Aphrodite"
(*the goddess of love, desire*) "is called Mylitta.
The woman follows the first man who throws
her the money, and repels no one. When
once she has accompanied him, and *has thereby satisfied the goddess*, she returns to her
home, and from thenceforth, however large
the sum offered to her, she will yield to no
one." Maspero declares that "this custom
still existed in the fifth century before our
era, and the Greeks who visited Babylon
about that time found it still in force." [61]

He also calls attention to the fact that "we
meet with a direct allusion to this same custom in the Bible, in the *Book of Baruch:* The
women, also, with cords about them, sitting
in the ways, burn bran for perfume; but if
any of them, drawn by some that passeth by,
lie with him, she reproacheth her fellow, that
she was not worthy of herself, nor her cord
broken. Ch. VI, verse 43."

Phallic rites and observances entered very

(61) Maspero (Sayce): *The Dawn of Civilization*, p. 640.

largely into the religion of the Assyrians, and
can be traced back, in some form or other,
even to the religion of the ancient Sumerians,
the root-stock from which the Chaldeans had
their origin.

In the third chapter of Hebrew history
according to Moses (Genesis III), we have an
unmistakable allusion to phallic worship in
the use of the serpent in the myth of man's
temptation and fall. The serpent was an
almost universal symbol of priapic adoration
throughout Egypt and Assyria; it achieved
this distinction, in all probability, from its
resemblance to the *instrumentum masculinum
generationis.** In a beautiful bronze plaque,
representing Nergal, the Chaldean god of
Hades, the *glans penis* of the god is distinctly
the head of the snake. A splendid drawing

(*) The author is fully aware of the fact that writers on
phallic worship ascribe other reasons for the adoption of the
snake as one of the chief symbols of the worship of the generative principle. He believes, however, that the primitive
originators of this cult were, psychically, too immature to
evolve any other than simple and objective ideas in regard to
this subject; hence he considers the above as the true origin
of this symbol.

of this plaque by Faucher-Gudin is given in
Maspero's *Dawn of Civilization.* [62] It may
be stated here that the uræus, or asp, which
was so prominently in evidence as one of the
principle signs of Egyptian royalty, was also
the symbol of the life-giving principle of Ra,
the sun-god.

Abraham, in all probability, instituted the
rite of circumcision in remembrance of the
Chaldean genital worship.* This sexual
fetichism was eminently religious in character
from its very inception among the ancient
Hebrews; yet Westermarck, in his *History
of Human Marriage,* considers this custom as
being of ornamental origin. [63] Now, it is
known beyond question of doubt that the
Hebrews and Abyssinians, who practiced this
rite, covered their nakedness, hence, it is folly

---

(62) *Op. cit.*, p. 691.

(*) Abraham was a Chaldean, and, in instituting circumcision, was undoubtedly influenced by the religious beliefs of
his people. Circumcision, however, was, with him, a new
and special phallic rite, and one not in vogue among the
Chaldeans. *Vid.* Genesis, 18:10.

(63) Westermarck: *History of Human Marriage,* p. 202 *et
seq.*

to suppose that they ornamented a portion of their bodies which always remained carefully hidden. Moreover, since it has been in use from very ancient times "among most of the tribes inhabiting the African West Coast, among all the Mohammedan peoples, among the Kafirs, among nearly all the peoples of Eastern Africa, among the Christian Abyssinians, Bogos, and Copts, throughout all the various tribes inhabiting Madagascar, and, in the heart of the Black Continent, among the Monbuttu and Akka; and since it is practiced very commonly in Australia, in many islands of Melanesia, in Polynesia, universally, in some parts of America, in Yucatan, on the Orinoco, and among certain tribes in Rio Branco in Brazil;" [64] and since most of these people wholly or partially hide their nakedness, it can not, necessarily, have had its origin in the desire for ornamentation. Again, since the rite of circumcision among these peo-

(64) Westermarck: *History of Human Marriage*, p. 201 *et seq*. See, also, Wallace: *Travels on the Amazon*, p. 117 *et seq*.

ples always takes place at puberty, when *vita
sexualis* begins, and is always accompanied by
other rites and ceremonies of deeply religious
significance, it must be a religious observance
and phallic in its nature. Girls, also, at,
puberty, among many tribes of Africa, among
certain races of the Malayan Archipelago and
South America have an operation performed
upon them. "*Sunt autem gentes, quarum con-
trarius mos est, ut clitoris et libia minora non
exsecentur, verum extendantur, et sæpe long-
issime extendantur.*" [65] Surely such a peculiar and uncalled-for performance has a deeper
significance than mere ornamentation, and
does not warrant the expression "*atque ista
etiam deformatio insigne pulchritudinis existi-
matur.*"

Tattooing, among certain races, is a phallic
rite, and in the Tahitians the priapic origin
of this procedure has been preserved in an
interesting myth. Hinæreeremonoi was the
daughter of the god and goddess Taaroa and

(65) Westermarck : *op. cit. ante*, p. 106.

Apouvaru. "As she grew up, in order to preserve her chasity, she was made *pahio*, or kept in a kind of inclosure, and constantly attended by her mother. Intent on her seduction, her brothers invented tattooing, and marked each other with the figure called Taomaro. Thus ornamented, they appeared before their sister, who admired the figures, and, in order to be tattooed herself, eluding the care of her mother, broke the inclosure that had been erected for her preservation, was tattooed, and became, also, the victim to the designs of her brothers. Tattooing thus originated among the gods, and was first practiced by the children of Taaroa, their principle deity. *In imitation of their example, and for the accomplishment of the same purposes it was practiced among men.*" * [66]

With very few exceptions, primitive peo-

(66) Ellis: *Polynesian Researches*, vol. i, p. 262; quoted, also, by Westermarck, *op. cit. ante.*, p. 179.

(*) After the ceremony of tattooing had been performed, the candidates were admitted to a religious society called *Areois*, which had for its object an "unrestrained and public abandonment to amorous pleasures." Letourneau: *The Evolution of Marriage*, p. 61.

ples, wherever found, have given or still give
unmistakable evidence of a knowledge of
phallic worship in some form or other. Many
of them still practice it, generally combined
with the religion from which it was evolved,
i. e., sun worship. The Ainu of Japan is a
notable example of a race whose religion
shows the presence of the elements of both
worships. The religion of this remarkable
people, notwithstanding the fact that it has
become decidedly ethical (they having arrived
at a knowledge of the good and evil principles),
yet show its sun birth.* Until very recently
the *couvade* existed in full force and vigor.
"As soon as a child was born, the father had
to consider himself very ill, and had, therefore,
to stay at home, wrapped up, by the fire. But
the wife, poor creature! had to stir about as
much and as quickly as possible. The idea
seems to have been that *life was passing from
the father into his child*." [67]

(*) Herodotus gives an interesting instance of the evolution
of phallic worship from nature worship. See *Clio*, 131.

(67) Batchelor: *The Ainu of Japan*, p. 44.

Among Slavonic races in early times, the
worship of the generative principle was almost universal. This continued, in a measure, even after the establishment of Christianity, and we find phallic rites masquerading
in the garb of Christian observances as late as
the sixteenth century in parts of Russia and
Hungary. Westermarck, in his chapter on
the human rut season in primitive times, says:
"Writers of the sixteenth century speak of
the existence of certain festivals in Russia, at
which great license prevailed. According to
Pamphil, these annual gatherings took place,
as a rule, at the end of June, the day before
the festival of St. John the Baptist, which in
pagan times was that of a divinity known by
the name of Jarilo, corresponding to the Priapus of the Greeks." [68] If my memory serves
me correctly, Wappäus says that a like festival was in existence among the Hungarians
two hundred years ago.[69] To this day cer-

---

(68) Westermarck : *The History of Human Marriage*, p. 30.
(69) Wappäus : *Allgem. Bevoelkerungsstatistik.*

tain religious sects of Russia and Hungary are in the habit of holding orgies at which all the ceremonics of the ancient Liberalia, Floralia, and Saturnalia are duplicated. These devotees claim that, when they have reached the acme of religious enthusiasm, the spirit of God directs them, hence their licentious and lustful acts can not be immoral.

When Great Britain was invaded and conquered by northern savages, the latter, unquestionably, introduced their own religious beliefs, which were largely phallic in character. The Teutonic god Fréa was the same as the Latin Priapus; while Friga, from whom our Friday gets its name, because this day was sacred to her, was the Teutonic Venus. Fréa is called Freyr in old Norse, and in old German, Fro.

Among the Swedes he was worshiped under the name of Fricco, and a statue of him at Upsala represented him in the characteristic attitude of the god of procreation. "*Tertius est Fricco, pacem voluptatemque largiens mortalibus, cujus etiam simulachrum fin-*

gunt ingcnti priapo." [70]   From this god a
vulgar word for copulation had its origin.
This word is in use to-day among the descendants of the Anglo-Saxons, thus proving that
the worship of the generative principle was
in vogue among our own immediate ancestors.

Statuettes of Priapus, bronzes representing
the sexual organs, and pottery covered with
phallic scenes have been found all over England.   These relics are remembrancers of the
Roman occupation when the worship of Priapus prevailed.   In the parish of Adel, Yorkshire, was found an altar erected to Priapus,
who seems to be called in this instance Men-
tula.   At this place were found many other
priapic relics, such as lamps, bracelets, amulets,
etc., etc. [71]   Several images of the triple phallus, as well as the single phallus, have been
brought to light in London; also phallic lamps,
bracelets, etc.

---

(70) Bremens: *De Situ Daniæ*, p. 23; quoted, also, by the
author of *The Worship of the Generative Powers,* p. 126.
(71) *The Worship of the Generative Powers*, p. 124.

All over England the Anglo-Saxon Fréa, or
Friga, has left remembrancers of his or her
worship in place-names. Fridaythorpe in
Yorkshire, and Friston (Fréa's stone), which
occurs in several parts of England, are examples. "We seem justified in supposing
that this and other names commencing with
the syllable Fri or Fry, are so many monuments
of the existence of phallic worship among our
Anglo-Saxon forefathers."[72] There are other
words in the English language which point
directly to this ancient religion; for instance,
fascinate and *fascination*. These words were
derived directly from the Latin word *fascinum*,
which was one of the names of the male organ
of generation. The fascinum was worn suspended from the necks of women, and was
supposed to possess magical powers; hence,
to *fascinate*. Horace makes use of the word
in Priapeia:

> "*Placet, Priape? Qui sunt arboris coma
> Sotes, sacrum revincte pampino caput,
> Ruber sedere cum rubente fascino.*"[73]

---

(72) *The Worship of the Generative Powers*, p. 127.
(73) Horace: *Priap. Carm.*, lxxxiv.

That the worship of the fascinum was in vogue during the eighth century * in Italy and in other countries under the religious jurisdiction of the Pope, the following from the *Judicia Sacerdotalia Criminibus*, clearly indicates : " If any one has performed incantation to the *fascinum*, or any incantation whatever, except one who chaunts the Creed or the Lord's Prayer, let him do penance on bread and water during three Lents." [74] During the ninth century the Council of Chalons promulgated a similar law, and in the twelfth century Buchardus repeats it, thus showing that the worship of the generative principle was continuous throughout that

(*) A well informed Jesuit priest once told me that several laws had been made about this time forbidding the worship of the female sexual organ, under the name of *abricot* or *apricot*. Rabelais used the word *abricot fendu* when speaking of the female genital organs. See his works. Was this term derived from the Biblical narrative of the genesis of the human race (the apple), or was it taken from the phallic symbol, the pomegranate? Did Moses get it from the Assyrians in the first place? I think he did.

(74) Martène and Durand : *Veterum Scriptorum Amplissima Collectio*, tom. vii, p. 35. *Si quis præcantaverit ad fascinum, vel qualescumque præcantationes excepto symbolum sanctum aut orationem dominicam qui cantat et cui cantatur, tres quadrigesimas in pane et aqua pœniteat.*

time.[75] That the worship of the fascinum
was in vogue as late as 1247 is proven by the
statutes of the Synod of Mans, which declare
that he who worships the fascinum shall be
seriously dealt with.[76]

In Scotland, as late as 1268, according to
the Chronicles of Lanercroft, the people were
in the habit of rubbing two pieces of wood
together until fire was produced. At the
same time an image of the phallus was elevated, and certain prayers were said to Priapus. This was the famous "need fire," and
was obtained in this way in order that it
might have the power of saving the cattle
from the plague. Need fire was produced in
this manner in the Highlands as late as 1356,
at which time a cattle plague ravaged the
country side. In Inverkeithing, a Catholic

(75) D. Burchardi: *Decretorum libri*, lib. x, c. 49.

(Some of these clerical references are taken from the
Worship of Priapus, but, since this work is exceedingly rare
and costly, and is not apt to come under the notice of the general reader, I have thought best to give the original authorities.)

(76) Martène and Durand: *Veterum Scriptorum Collectio
Amplissima*, tom. vii, col. 1377.

priest gathered all the young girls of the village and made them dance around a statue of Priapus. He himself led the dance, carrying a large wooden image of the phallus, and excited these medieval bacchantes to licentious movements and actions by his own actions and language.

When called to account by his bishop, he excused his action by stating that such performances were common in his parish. These phallic observances occurred in Easter week, March 29 – April 15, 1282.[77]

In Ireland, the female sexual organs seem to have been the symbol of phallic worship most in use. In the arches over the doorways of churches, a female figure, with the person fully exposed, was invariably so placed that the external organs of generation at once caught the eye. These figures were called *Shela-na-gig*, which in Irish means "Julian the giddy." Sometimes these images were placed on the walls and used as caryatides.

(77) *The Chronicles of Lanercroft.*

From this symbol the horseshoe's power to
ward off evil and bring good luck has been
evolved. The people in olden times were in
the habit of painting, or sketching with char-
coal, drawings of the female genitalia over the
doors of their houses to ward off bad luck.
These drawings were necessarily rude, and
probably resembled a horseshoe more than
they did the object for which they were in-
tended. In course of time, when the symbol
had lost its original significance, the horseshoe entirely took the place of the phallic
image.

Herodotus says that Sesostris, king of
Egypt, was in the habit of erecting pillars in
the countries conquered by his armies, on
which he had the female genitals engraved in
order to show his contempt.[78] I think that
the historian misinterprets the meaning of the
pillars; the Egyptians were phallic worshipers, and these obelisks were, in all probability,
altars to Priapus.

---

(78) Herodotus: *Euterpe*, 102.

The beneficent influence of this particular phallic symbol has been well brought out in several classical stories. When Ceres was wandering over the world in her search after Proserpine, she came to the house of a peasant woman, Baubo by name. Baubo saw that the goddess was heart-sick and miserable, so she offered her a drink of cyceon (κυκεων). The goddess refused the refreshing mixture, and continued her lamentations. Fully believing in the virtue and efficacy of the symbol, Baubo lifted her robe and showed Ceres her genitals.* The goddess burst into laughter and at once drank the cyceon.[79] The same superstition appears in a celebrated book of the sixteenth century, *Le Moyen de Parvenir*. The author of the " Worship of the Generative Powers " gives the following instructive extract from this work:

Hermès. On nomme ainsi ceux qui n'ont point vu le con de leur femme ou de leur garce.

(*) For an analogous ceremony, see Herodotus, *Euterpe*, 60.
(79) Arnobius: *Adversus Gentes*, lib. v, c. 5.

*Le pauvre valet de chez nous n'étoit donc pas
coquebin ; il eut beau le voir.*

Varro.   Quand ?

*Hermès. Attendez, étant en fiançailles, il vou-
loit prendre le cas de sa fiancée ; elle ne le vouloit
pas : il faisoit le malade, et elle lui demandoit :
" Qu'y a-t-il, mon ami ?"   " Hélas, ma mie, je
suis si malade, que je n'en puis plus ; je mour-
rai si je ne vois ton cas."   " Vraiment voire ?"
dit-elle.   " Hélas ! oui, si je l'avois vu, je guéri-
rois."   Elle ne lui voulut point montrer ; à la
fin, ils furent mariés.   Il advint, trois ou quatre
mois après, qu'il fut fort malade ; et il envoya sa
femme au médicin pour porter de son eau.   En
allant, elle s'avisa de ce qu'il lui avoit dit en
fiançailles.   Elle retourna vitement, et se vint
mettre sur le lit ; puis, levant cotte et chemise lui
présenta son cela en belle vue, et lui disoit :
" Jean, regarde le con, et te guéris."* [80]

Sir William Hamilton writes to Richard
Payne Knight from Naples in the year 1781,
as follows :

" Having last year made a curious discovery,

---

(80) *The Worship of the Generative Powers*, p. 185.

that in a province of this kingdom, not fifty miles from its capital, a sort of devotion is still paid to Priapus, the obscene divinity of the ancients (though under another denomination), I have thought it a circumstance worth recording; particularly as it offers a fresh proof of the similitude of the Popish and Pagan religion, so well observed by Dr. Middleton in his celebrated Letter from Rome; therefore I mean to deposit the authentic proofs of this assertion in the British Museum when a proper opportunity shall offer." Sir William goes on to relate how he found many phallic amulets, charms, etc., in the possession of the people, and then describes the votive offerings laid upon the altar at a feast given in honor of Saints Cosmus and Damianus, in a church called by their names. The offerings were waxen images of the phallus. "The vows are chiefly presented by the female sex," continues he, "and they are seldom such as represent legs, arms, etc., but most commonly the male parts of generation. A person who was at this fête in the year 1780, told me that he heard a woman say, at the time she presented a vow, ' *Santo Cosimo benedetto, cosi lo voglio.*' " [81]

This church was in Isernia, a little village about fifty miles from Naples, and away from the direct line of travel, hence its inhabitants saw little of the world, and therefore kept to their old customs longer than their more favored neighbors. Thus it happened that, even in the latter half of the eighteenth century, Priapus had his votaries almost within the shadow of the Vatican! These phallic rites were finally abolished by episcopal command.

One of the most common amulets or charms against *jettitura*, or the " evil eye," the *bête noire* of every Italian, is a little coral hand. The middle finger of this hand is extended, thus representing the penis, while the other fingers are closed on the palm, thus representing the testicles. In ancient times, when a man extended his hand, closed in this manner, it was

---

(81) Knight: *The Worship of Priapus*, pp. 3-6, 7.

a gesture of insult and anger; to-day this gesture is only made in derision and contempt. The hand closed in this way, or, rather, with the thumb projecting between the first and second fingers (another very common phallic symbol or sign), was called a "fig;" hence, the old expression of contempt and indifference, "a fico for you, sir," now modernized into "I don't care a fig."

France, as well as Italy, had her phallic charms and her phallic saints. Priapus was a god to the ancients—to the people of the Middle Ages he was a saint. According to M. Dulaure, in the south of France, Provence, Languedoc, and the Lyonnais, he was worshiped under the name of St. Foutin. This name is derived from that of the first bishop of Lyons, Fotinus, to whom the people had transferred (as they have done to many other sainted individuals) the distinguishing characteristics of a god; in this instance, Priapus. At Lyons there was an immense wooden phallus, and the women were in the habit of

6

scraping this image, and then steeping the wood-dust in water, which they drank as a remedy against barrenness. Sometimes they gave it to the men in order to stimulate sexuality or sensuality. At Varailles, in Provence, waxen images of the male and female sexual organs were offered to St. Foutin, and, since these images were suspended from the ceiling and moved by every vagrant current of air, the effect was sometimes very astonishing. "*Témoin Saint Foutin de Varailles en Provence, auquel sont dédiées les parties honteuses de l'un et de l'autre sexe, formées en cire; le plancher de la chapelle en est fort garni, et, quand le vent les fait entrebattre, cela débauche un peu les dévotions à l'honneur de ce Saint.*"[82]

This worship at Varailles was identical with that of Isernia; the votive offerings were waxen images or models of the genital organs, while the saints differed only in name, not in character. At Embrun the worship of St. Foutin was a little different. The women at

---

(82) L'Estolle: *Confession de Sancy*, pp. 383, 391.

this last mentioned place poured wine on the phallus; this wine was collected in a bucket, and, when it became sour, it was used as a medicine for barrenness.

When Embrun was besieged and taken by the Protestants in 1585, this phallus was found among the other sacred relics, and its head " was red with the wine which had been poured upon it." [83]   In the church of St. Eutropius, at Orange, a large phallus covered with leather was seized and burnt by the Protestants in 1562. Dulaure says that the sexual organs were objects of worship at Porigny, Viviers, Vendre in the Bourbonnais, Cives, Auxerre, Puy-en-Velay, and at hundreds of other places. Some of these phalli were recreated as fast as they were worn away by zealous devotees. They were so arranged in the walls of the churches that, " as the phallic end in front be- came shortened (by scrapings), a blow from a mallet from behind thrust it forward, so that it was restored to its original length." [84]

(83) *The Worship of Priapus*, p. 141.
(84) *Ibid.*

/ 𝑛𝑙 —

In the public square of Batavia there was formerly kept a bronze canon which had been captured from the natives. The touch-hole of this piece of ordnance was made in the shape of a phallic hand or " fig," which I have described elsewhere. The barren Malay women were in the habit of seating themselves on this hand in order that they might become pregnant.* An analogous custom was prevalent in France and elsewhere in Europe during the Middle Ages. This habit led to sexual abuses, and was finally condemned by the ecclesiastical authorities. Indeed, the Church inflicted severe penances on the women who were guilty of using phalli : " *Mulier qualique molimine aut*

(*) According to Abel de Rémusat (*Nouv. Mel. Asiatiques*, p. 116), the custom of *Ichin-than*, or religious defloration, was formerly in use in Cambodia and Malabar. This custom seems to be analogous to the *jus primæ noctis*, as practiced by many tribes, where the woman, on her bridal night, has to yield herself up to the male marriage guests—*jus primæ noctis*, as thus practiced, must not be confounded with the seignorial right, the right of the lord, or ruler. The former right is regarded in the light of a *quasi* religious observance, while the latter is not. The former was in vogue in ancient times in the Balearic Isles and among the ancient Peruvians; recently among several aboriginal tribes of India, in Burmah, in Cashmere, in Madagascar, in Arabia, and in New Zealand. Vid. Teulon : *Orig. de la Famille*, p. 69.

se ipsam aut cum altera fornicans tres annos pœ-niteat, unum ex his pane et aqua. Cum sancti-moniali per machinam fornicans, annos septem pœniteat, duos ex his in pane et aqua." [85] We see by this that nuns were more severely punished than were other women.

This use of the phallus is mentioned in the Bible, where it is bitterly condemned by one of the prophets : "Thou hast also taken thy fair jewels of my gold and of my silver, which I had given thee, and madest to thyself images of men, and didst commit whoredom with them." [86] Finally, it was the custom of the young girls of France during the Middle Ages (like the maidens of certain savage races), who were on the eve of marriage, to offer up to St. Foutin their last maiden robes. From the evidence here adduced, we see that phallic worship existed in some parts of Europe as late as the latter half of the eighteenth century, and that it was almost universal during

(85) Martène et Durand: *Coll. Antiq. Can. Pœnit.*, iv, 52.
(86) *Ezekiel*: chap. xvi, v. 17.

the Middle Ages. According to Becan, [87]
Golnitz, [88] and other historians, there were
several other phallic saints besides St. Foutin
who were worshiped in Belgium, Spain, Germany and other European countries; but,
since their adoration was similar to that of St.
Foutin, I do not think it necessary to give a
description of it here. It has been shown
conclusively that worship of the generative
principle was in vogue among the Latins, the
Greeks, the ancient Germans, the Saxons, the
Danes, the Gauls, the Iberians, the Picts, the
Celts and the Britons. It has been demonstrated, also, that vestiges of phallic worship
existed in England, France, Italy, Spain and
Germany during the Middle Ages. ' As late
as the latter part of the eighteenth century
wax images of the phallus were used as votive
offerings in the town of Isernia, not many
miles from Genoa; the beribboned May-
pole of our May-day festival is but the

(87) Becan: *Origines Antwerpianæ*, lib. 1, pp. 26, 101.
(88) Golnitz: *Itinerarium Belgico-Gallicum*, p. 52.

flower decked phallus of the Roman matrons;
charms against *jettitura,* "the evil eye,"
little coral hands with the middle finger
extended (in ancient days one of the most
common symbols of Priapus) can still be pur-
chased in the streets of Rome. "This worship" (that of Priapus) "which was but part
of that of the generative powers, appears to
have been the most ancient of the supersti-
tions of the human race, and has prevailed
more or less among all known peoples before
the introduction of Christianity; and, singu-
larly enough, *so deeply it seems to have been
implanted in human nature* that even the pro-
mulgation of the gospel did not abolish it, for
it continued to exist, accepted and often encouraged by the medieval clergy." [89]

So very ancient was the inception of the
worship of the generative principle that we
have some reason for believing that even the
cave-dwellers practiced this cult. It was stated
in the *Moniteur,* January, 1865, that "in the

(89) Knight: *op. cit. ante,* p. 117.

province of Venice, in Italy, excavations in a bone-cave have brought to light, beneath ten feet of stalagmite, bones of animals, mostly post-tertiary, of the usual description found in such places, flint implements, with a needle of bone having an eye and point, and a plate of argillaceous compound, on which was scratched a rude drawing of the phallus."[90] Thus we see that, possibly, from the time of the cave-dwellers to almost the beginning of the nineteenth century, phallic worship existed in Southern Europe! From the Sagas, folk-lore tales, and myths of the Norse we have every reason for believing that it existed for almost as great a length of time in Northern Europe. That in Western Europe, before and during the Middle Ages, it flourished in a variety of forms, we have unimpeachable testimony.

In this brief outline of phallic worship I have endeavored to show that the worship of the generative principle has been universal;

---

(90) *The Worship of the Generative Powers*, foot-note p. 117.

that it is still practiced by primitive peoples, and that vestiges of it lingered among
certain civilized peoples until, comparatively
speaking, a recent time. In order to show what
a height of idealization and abstraction it
had reached at a time when Greece stood at
the head of the civilized world, I will close
this part of my essay with the following quotation from Knight's strong, erudite, and
exhaustive treatise : " The ancient theologists
. . . finding that they could conceive no
idea of infinity, were content to revere the
Infinite Being in the most general and efficient
exertion of his power — attraction; whose
agency is perceptible through all matter, and
to which all motion may, perhaps, be ulti-
mately traced. His agency being supposed
to extend through the whole material world,
and to produce all the various revolutions by
which its system is sustained, his attributes
were, of course, extremely numerous and
varied. These were expressed by various
titles and epithets in the mystic hymns and

litanies, which the artists endeavored to represent by various forms and characters of men and animals. The great characteristic attribute was represented by the organ of generation in that state of tension and rigidity which is necessary to the due performance of its functions. Many small images of this kind have been found among the ruins of Herculaneum and Pompeii, attached to bracelets, which the chaste and pious matrons of antiquity wore round their necks and arms. In these the organ of generation appears alone, or accompanied by the wings of incubation, in order to show that the wearer devoted herself wholly and solely to procreation, the great end for which she was ordained. So expressive a symbol, being constantly in view, must keep her attention fixed on its natural object, and continually remind her of the gratitude she owed the Creator for having taken her into his service, made her partaker of his most valuable blessings, and employed her as the passive instrument in the exertion of his most beneficial power. The female organs of generation were revered as symbols of the generative power of nature or matter, as the male's were of the generative powers of God." [91]

---

(91) Knight: *The Worship of Priapus*, p. 27 *et seq.*

PART III.

The Correlation of Religious Emotion and Sexual Desire.

That there exists a relationship between the cultivated ethical emotion, religious feeling, and the essentially natural physio-psychical function, sexual desire or *libido*, is a fact noticed and commented on by many thinkers and writers. The literature of the subject is, however, exceedingly fragmentary and disconnected, no author (as far as I have been able to determine) having devoted as much as one thousand words to the consideration of this very interesting psychical phenomenon. Hence, my data have been gathered from many sources, which are as diversified as they are numerous.

Beyond a question of doubt, man becomes religiously enthused most frequently either early in life, when pubescence is, or is about to be, established, or late in life, when sexual desire has become either entirely extinct or very much abated. Young boys and girls are exceedingly impressionable at, or just before, puberty, and are apt to embrace religion with the utmost enthusiasm. A distinguished evangelist declares that "men and women seldom or never enter into the kingdom of God after they have arrived at maturity. Out of a thousand converts, seven hundred are converted before they are twenty years old." [92]

The Roman Catholic church is keenly alive to these facts, therefore requires the rite of confirmation to be administered, if possible, to its would-be communicants at, or before, the age of puberty.

Of all the insanities of the pubescent state, erotomania and religious mania are the most frequent and the most pronounced. Sometimes they go hand in hand, the most inordinate sensuality being coupled with abnor-

(92) B. Fay Mills, *Sermon to Young Men and Young Women*, at Owensboro, Ky., May 20, 1894.

mal religious zeal. A young woman of my acquaintance, whose conduct has given rise to much scandal, is, at times, a reincarnate Messalina, while at other times she is the very embodiment of ethical and religious purity. Another young girl, in whom *vita sexualis* was about to be established, became religiously insane and had delusions in which she declared that she was in heaven and sitting at the right hand of God. She declared this over and over again, while shamelessly committing manustrupation! Krafft-Ebing calls attention to this relation between religious and sexual feeling in psycho-pathological states. "It suffices," says he, "to recall how intense sensuality makes itself manifest in the clinical history of many religious maniacs; the motley mixture of religious and sexual delusions that is so frequently observed in psychoses (*e. g.*, in maniacal women who think they are or will be the mother of God), but particularly in masturbatic insanity; and finally, the sexual, cruel self-punishment, injuries, self-castrations, and even self-crucifixions, resulting from abnormal religio-sexual feeling." [93]

An example of the last mentioned self-immolation (self-crucifixion) is given by Berghierri, and is a remarkable instance of the interchangeableness of religious emotion and sexual desire in psychopathic individuals. The man in question, who had been intensely sensual, manufactured a cross, nailed himself to it, and ingeniously managed to suspend himself and cross from the window of his sleeping apartment.

"All through the history of insanity the student has occasion to observe this close alliance of sexual and religious ideas; an alliance which may be partly accounted for because of the prominence which sexual themes have in most creeds, as illustrated in ancient times by the phallus worship of the Egyptians, the ceremonies of the Friga cultus of the Saxons, the frequent and detailed reference to sexual topics in the Koran and several other books

(93) Kraft-Ebing, *Psychopathia Sexualis*, p. 8.

of the kind, and which is further illustrated
in the performances which, to come down to
a modern period, characterize the religious
revival and camp-meeting as they tinctured
their medieval model, the Münster Anabap-
tist movement." [94]

Not only is this alliance shown in diseased
states, but it is also in evidence in normal,
healthy conditions. In this age of civilization, youth, hedged about as it is by certain
moral restrictions, and carnally ignorant of
the differences of the sexes, at the dawn
of sexual life, filled as it is with indefinite
longings and desires, eagerly seizes upon religion to satisfy its yearnings. And, strange as
it may seem, this substitution of a cultivated
ethical emotion for a natural desire is, in the
vast majority of instances, entirely successful.

Men, owing to their greater freedom, soon
learn the difference of the sexes and the delights of sexual congress; women, hedged in
by conventionalities and deterred by their

---

(94) Spitzka: *Insanity*, p. 39.

innate passivity, remain, for the most part, in ignorance of sexual knowledge until their marriage. For this reason it happens that very many more women than men experience religious emotion. *Young married men and women, who are in perfect sexual health, and who have not experienced religion before marriage, seldom give this emotion a single thought until late in life, when both libido and vita sexualis are on the wane or are extinct.* Voltaire cynically, though truthfully, observes that when woman is no longer pleasing to man she then turns to God. A woman who has been disappointed in love almost invariably seeks consolation in religion. The virtuous unmarried woman, who has been unsuccessful in the pursuit of a husband, invariably turns to God and religion with impassioned zeal and energy.

Ungratified, or, rather, *unsatisfied,* sensuality very frequently gives rise to great religio-sexual enthusiasm. The circumcised foreskin of Christ, where it was and what had become of

7

it, was a source of continual worriment to the
nun Blanbekin; in an ecstacy of ungratified
libido, St. Catherine of Genoa would frequently
cast herself on the hard floor of her cell, crying: "Love! love! I can endure it no
longer;" St. Armelle and St. Elizabeth were
troubled with *libido* for the child Jesus; [95] an
old prayer is quite significant: "Oh, that I had
found thee, Holy Emanuel; *Oh, that I had
thee in my bed to bring delight to body and soul!*
Come and be mine, and my heart shall be thy
resting-place." [96]   Francis Parkman calls attention to the fact that the nuns sent over to
America in colonization days were frequently
seized with religio-sexual frenzy. "She heard,"
writes he of Marie de l'Incarnation, "in a
trance, a miraculous voice. It was that of
Christ, promising to become her spouse.
Months and years passed, full of troubled
hopes and fears, when again the voice sounded
in her ear, with assurance that the promise

(95) Kraft-Ebing: *op. cit. ante,* p. 8, foot-note.
(96) *Ibid.*

was fulfilled, and that she was, indeed, his
bride. Now ensued phenomena which are not
infrequent among Roman Catholic female
devotees, when unmarried, or married unhap-
pily, and *which have their source in the necessi-
ties of a woman's nature.*" (The italics are my
own.) "To her excited thought, her divine
spouse became a living presence; and her language to him, as recorded by herself, is of
intense passion. She went to prayer, agitated
and tremulous, as if to a meeting with an
earthly lover. 'Oh, my Love,' she exclaimed,
'when shall I embrace you? Have you no
pity on the torments that I suffer? Alas! alas!
my Love, my Beauty, my Life! Instead of
healing my pain, you take pleasure in it.
Come, let me embrace you, and die in your
sacred arms!'"[97] The historian remarks
that the "holy widow," as her biographers

---

(97) Francis Parkman: *The Jesuits in North America*, p. 175.
"*O amour, quand vous embrasserai-je? N'avez vous point pitie
de moi dans le tourment que je souffre? Hélas! mon amour, ma
beauté, ma vie! au lieu de me guerir, vous vous plaisez à mes maux.
Venez donc que je vous embrasse et je meure entre vos bras sacres.*"
Journal de Marie de l'Incarnation.

call her, is an example, and a lamentable one, of the tendency of the erotic principle to ally itself with high religious excitement and enthusiasm. Further along he says that "some of the pupils of Marie de l'Incarnation, also, had mystical marriages with Christ; and the impassioned rhapsodies of one of them being overheard, she nearly lost her character, as it was thought that she was apostrophizing an earthly lover." [98]

The instances of religio-sexual outbursts in nuns and Roman Catholic female devotees who lead celibate lives are very numerous; I will, however, call attention to but one other: St. Veronica was so much in love with the divine lion that she took a young lion to bed with her, fondled and kissed it, and allowed it to suck her breasts. [99] Throughout sacred literature, beginning with the Bible itself, religio-sexual feeling is very much *en*

---

(98) Francis Parkman : *The Jesuits in North America*, p. 176.
(99) Friedreich : *Psychologie*, p. 389.

evidence. Hosea married a prostitute because —so he declared—God commanded him so to do. If Solomon's beautiful song is typical of the Church and the Christ (as some theologians teach), then it is an unmistakable instance of religio-sexual feeling; religious emotion and sexual desire walk hand in hand through the measures of this impassioned verse. Circumcision, now eminently a religious ceremony, is, unquestionably, a sexual fetich and a phallic rite, which has been handed down from antiquity, when all the world were phallic worshipers! The very pillars set up by the patriarchs in commemoration of certain events were but rude images of the phallus, while not a few of the mysteries of the Holy of Holies itself were but vestiges of Chaldean and Egyptian genital worship!

That a relationship between, and an interchangeableness of, these two widely dissimilar psychcial operations, *i. e.*, religious emotion and sexual desire, does exist, there can be no doubt.* Now, what is the cause of, the reason for, this relationship? Mantegazza, Maudsley, Schleiermacher, Krafft-Ebing, and many others have endeavored, incidentally, to assign reasons for this relationship, but have, in my opinion, signally failed. Spitzka has tentatively, and without elaborating his idea in the least, suggested a theory which, I believe, solves the problem in every essential point. Says he in "Insanity," page 39: This "alliance" (between religious emotion and *libido*) "may be partly accounted for because of the prominence which sexual themes have in most creeds, as illustrated in ancient times by the phallus worship of the Egyptians, the ceremonies of the Friga cultus of the Saxons, the frequent and detailed reference to sexual topics in the Koran and several other books of the kind, etc." Dr. Spitzka does not enter into any discussion of the matter; he simply

*The author believes that upon the correlation of religious emotion and sexual desire depends, in a great measure, the stability of sexual morality. Were it not for this correlation, sexual promiscuity would be the rule throughout the world.

asserts his belief in the cause of the relationship, and then dismisses the subject without further comment.

Now, permit me, as briefly as possible, to designate the cause of the relationship between, and the interchangeableness of, religious feeling and sexual desire, which, as I believe, is to be found in the once wide-spread existence of phallic worship.

Some ten or twelve years ago, in an article on Suicide, which was published in the *American Practitioner and News*, I suggested (as a possible explanation for certain psychical phenomena) the existence in man of two consciousnesses, an active, vigilant consciousness and a pseudo-dormant consciousness. Again, in the *American Naturalist*, in an essay entitled "The Psychology of Hypnotism,"[100] I reasserted this theory and, to a certain extent, elaborated it. I placed man's active consciousness in the cortical portion of the brain, and his pseudo-dormant, *unconscious* consciousness

(100) *Loc. cit.*, November, 1894.

(arbitrarily, be it confessed) in the basilar ganglia, and called this latter consciousness, "ganglionic consciousness."

Recently, much has been written on the doctrine of duplex personality, notably by Mr. F. W. H. Myers, in a series of papers read before the Society of Psychical Research. Prof. Newbold has also written very entertainingly and instructively on this subject. While not fully accepting the theory of "duplex personality," *i. e.*, active consciousness and *subliminal consciousness* (Myers' name for the pseudo-dormant consciousness), as having been proven, Newbold says: "Of all the theories developed from the point of independence, Mr. Myers' is the most comprehensive in its scope, is kept in most constant touch with what the author regards as facts, and displays the greatest philosophic insight."[101] According to the theory of duplex personality, many instincts, desires, and emotions have been

(101) Newbold: *Appleton's Popular Science Monthly*, February, 1897, p. 516.

crowded out of the active consciousness and have been relegated to the pseudo-dormant consciousness. This has been brought about by a "process of selection out of an infinity of possible elements solely on the grounds of utility." Thus the *cause* for our horror of incest is hidden away in our subliminal consciousness; yet we can not but think, with Westermarck, that this instinct is but the result of natural selection,[102] the utility of the factor or factors occasioning it being no longer in evidence or required. Again, at certain seasons, man is seized with *waldliebe* (forest-love) and longs to flee from the haunts of men, and, with gun and rod, to revert, as far as possible, to the state of his savage ancestors. The desire is safely hidden away in his subliminal consciousness until favoring circumstances tempt it forth. It is not alone in "sleep, dreams, hypnosis, trance, and ecstacy that we see a temporary subsidence of the upper consciousness and the upheaval of a

(102) Westermarck : *History of Human Marriage*, p. 352.

subliminal stratum"; there are many other
states and many other causes for this strange
psychical phenomenon.

I have demonstrated in the preceding pages
that the worship of the generative principle
was almost, if not wholly, universal; I have
also shown that the beliefs, rites, and ceremonies of this cult made a lasting impression
upon the minds of every people among whom
it gained a foothold. Take the case of the
ancient Hebrews. Notwithstanding the fact
that they were tried in the furnace of Javeh's
awful wrath time and again; notwithstanding the fact that famine, pestilence, war, and
imprisonment destroyed them by thousands;
and, notwithstanding the fact that they were
threatened with utter and absolute annihilation—all on account of this cult—they would
not wholly abandon it. The words of the
prophets become almost pathetic as we read,
over and over again, that, although the kings
did that which was pleasing in the sight of the
Lord, " the high places and the groves were

not destroyed." Take the case of the Aztecs.
Crushed beneath the iron heels of Spain's
hardy buccaneers, an utterly broken and conquered race, Cortes turned them over to the
ministering care of his zealous priests. The
prison, agonizing torture, and the awful stake
succeeded, at last, in Christianizing them;
they became children of Holy Mother Church!
And yet, hundreds of years after this "glori-
ous victory of the cross," Biart finds the
humble offerings of their descendants at the
feet of Mictlanteuctli! The modern Christian
Indian, in the deep shadows of the night,
steals forth to offer up in secrecy a prayer at
the feet of one of the phallic trinity! What
matters it to the modern Aztec that his peti-
tion is offered to the ruler of Mictlan, the hell
of his forefathers, instead of to the mighty
Ipalnemoani, the Life-Giver?[103]   In his
opinion, Mictlanteuctli represents the entire
Aztec theogony, for has not his white priest
kept the name of *this* god green in his mem-

(103) Biart: *The Aztecs*, p. 110.

ory? All the other gods have been forgotten; their personalities have been absorbed
into that of the god of hell, for he has had
advertisers in the shape of Catholic priests
ever since the fall of the Aztec Empire! Take
the case of the Peruvians. Although the
Place of Gold and the beautiful Virgins of the
Sun are not even memories to the decendants
of the Incas, the religion which gave rise to
them is not wholly forgotten; "phallic rites
and ceremonies are to be observed interwoven
with their Christian ritual and belief!" Take
the case of the Roman Catholic devotees of
Isernia, of Varailles, of Lyons, of hundreds
of other places during the latter half of the
eighteenth century. Priapus died when the
first Christian emperor took his seat on the
throne of Imperial Rome, and yet, hundreds
and hundreds of years thereafter, we behold
some of the mysteries of Eleusis almost within
the shadow of St. Peter's!

Now, why is this? There can be but one
answer, and that is that these people simply

RELIGION AND LUST. 109

inherited a portion of the *psychos* of their forefathers, which made the tenets of this religion natural and easy of belief. I have demonstrated, I believe, that religious feeling was not a psychical trait in the beginning; like a number of other mental attributes, it was the result of evolution.[104] Mental abstraction, especially as associated with religious feeling, was the result of psychical growth, of psychically inherited experiences. As *psychos* grew beneath the fostering influence of ages of experience, the mind became able to formulate abstract thought. In the beginning, the process of ratiocination was, necessarily, very simple; but, simple as it was, it was able to recognize the source of life—first, in the sun, then, in the second place, in man himself;

---

(104) Huxley: *Essays;* Haeckel: *The History of Creation;* Haeckel: *The Evolution of Man;* Peschel: *The Races of Man;* De Quatrefages: *The Human Species;* Draper: *The Conflict Between Religion and Science;* White: *History of the Warfare of Science with Theology;* Romanes: *Mental Evolution in Man;* Wallace: *The Malay Archipelago (The Races of Man in the Malay Archipelago,* c. xl); Darwin's *Works;* Maudsley: *The Physiology of Mind;* Tylor: *Anthropology;* Spencer: *Synthetic Philosophy—Prin. Psych., Prin. Sociol.*

and, finally and *abstractly*, in a source outside
of, but connected with, man. This abstract
source, which sprung from sexuality, *ab initio*,
they deified and worshiped. Thus we see
that, in the very beginning, the worship of the
generative principle sprung from, and was a
part of, man himself. Throughout thousands
and thousands of years, religious feeling and
sexual desire, the component parts of phallic
adoration, were intimately associated; finally,
religio-sexuality became an instinct, just as a
belief in the existence of a double or soul became an instinct.

Belief in the existence of a soul has never
been repressed; its utility is still recognized;
hence, it is present in our active consciousness.
The accumulated experiences of civilization
have, however, declared the inutility of phallic
worship, hence, it has been crowded out of our
active consciousness by a process of selection
and has been relegated to the innermost recesses of our subliminal consciousness, where
also dwell many other formerly active instincts

of our savage ancestors. When circumstances favoring their appearances occur, these pseudo-dormant instincts always become evident; it is due to this fact that the correlation of religious emotion and sexual desire exists.

PSYCHICAL PROBLEMS.

THE PSYCHOLOGY OF HYPNOTISM.

The various phenomena accompanying animal magnetism, so-called, have been observed
and commented on by man since a very early
era in his history. Our savage ancestors,
whose psychical development had just begun,
considered these manifestations to be a direct
evidence of the supernatural, and those individuals who, either actively or passively, gave
evidences of this, to them, occult power, to be
directly influenced by supernatural agencies.
This manner of regarding these phenomena
has, in a measure, descended to us, and the
vast majority of civilized beings of to-day
look with a certain awe on the person who is
laboring under hypnotic influence. The skep-
tical minority, however, generally regard hypnotism as a baseless fraud and imposture.
Both classes of individuals are in error; the
first because there is nothing supernatural in
the phenomena of so-called animal magnetism ;

the second because these phenomena really do
exist and are the result of perfectly natural
causes. The term, animal magnetism, owes
its origin to a tradition which came into existence about the middle of the sixteenth century. At that time man conceived the idea
that he could influence his fellows in a manner
analogous to that of a magnet, attracting some
and repelling others. The first written evidence of this belief occurs in the work of
Paracelsus. He maintained that "the human
body was endowed with a double magnetism,
that one portion attracted to itself the planets,
and was nourished by them, whence came
wisdom, thought, and the senses; that the
other portion attracted to itself the elements
and disintegrated them, whence came flesh
and blood; that the attractive and hidden
virtue of man resembles that of amber and
the magnet; that by this virtue, the magnetic virtue of healthy persons attracts the
enfeebled magnetism of those who are sick."
The latter part of this doctrine is believed by

many people at the present time; witness the widespread belief that an enfeebled person should not occupy the same bed with a strong, lusty individual, lest the enfeebled vitality of the one should be overcome and be absorbed by the stronger vitality of the other. Many scientists of the sixteenth and seventeenth centuries, notably Glocenius, Fludd, Kircher, Burgrave, and Maxwell, accepted the doctrines of Paracelsus, and declared that all natural phenomena could be explained through magnetism. These learned gentlemen thought that by magnetizing talismans and hanging them about the persons of the sick the vital spirit could be infused thence into the bodies of invalids, thus effecting cures.

Anthony Mesmer, who was born in Germany in 1734, discarded the talismans and magical boxes of his predecessors, and applied this so-called universal principle directly to the bodies of the sick through the agency of passes and contact. In the beginning of his career, however, Mesmer used the magnetic steel tractors of the Jesuit, Father Hell. But he soon abandoned them and confined himself to manual manipulations and passes, asserting that animal magnetism was entirely distinct from the influence exerted by the magnet.

In 1779 Mesmer left Vienna and came to Paris, where he at once began to give lectures on his theory of the magnetic fluid. In these lectures he declared that " he had discovered a principle capable of curing all diseases." Say Binet and Feré: " He summed up his theory in twenty-seven propositions, or, rather, assertions, most of which only reproduce the cloudy conceptions of magnetic medicine." These propositions, while they are full of the mysticism, the errors, and the superstition naturally belonging to the period at which they were formulated, yet contain the germs of scientific truths. As I wish to establish, later on in this paper, the fact that some individuals are more susceptible to hypnotic influence than are others, I will here introduce evidence obtained from the writings of one who witnessed Mesmer's *séances*. Says Bailly: . . . "They are so submissive to the magnetizer that even when they appear to be in a stupor, his voice, a glance, or sign will rouse them from it. It is impossible not to admit from all these results, that some great force acts upon and masters the patients, and that this force appears to reside in the magnetizer. It has been observed that *many women* and *few men* are subject to such crises." These crises were characterized by " *convulsions, cries, shouts, and groans.*" The same writer says elsewhere: "It has been likewise observed that they (crises) are only established after the lapse of two or three hours, and that when one is established others soon and *successively* begin." (Certain words and expressions are here and elsewhere italicized for future reference.) Mesmer's treatment became exceedingly popular. He consequently incurred the jealousy and hatred of the Academy of Science and the Academy of Medicine, these academies emphatically declaring that there was nothing in his method

and that his theory was arrant nonsense.
Whereupon Mesmer left France, notwithstanding the fact that the government offered
him a life-pension of 20,000 francs on the sole
condition of his remaining and continuing his
method of practice. He returned, however,
at the solicitation of his admirers, who offered
him a purse of 10,000 louis for a series of lectures on magnetism. These lectures were
published and set the kingdom into a ferment,
many declaring that Mesmer was a charlatan
and a fraud, while as many more declared that
he was a great discoverer and a benefactor of
the human race. In 1784 the government or-
dered an investigation and appointed a commission to inquire into magnetism. Their
report is exceeding interesting, inasmuch as
it shows how very near, indeed, these men
of wisdom were, in grasping the salient
features of hypnotism. Benjamin Franklin
was a member of this commission, his name
being signed first of all. A translation of
their report reads as follows: "The com-

missioners have ascertained that the animal magnetic fluid is not perceptible by any of the senses; that it has no action either on themselves or the patients subjected to it. They are convinced that pressure and contact effect changes which are rarely favorable to the animal system, and which injuriously affect the imagination. Finally, they have demonstrated, by decisive experiments, that imagination, apart from magnetism, produces convulsions, and that *magnetism without imagination produces nothing.* They have come to the unanimous conclusion, with respect to the existence and utility of magnetism, that there is nothing to prove the existence of animal magnetic fluid; that this fluid, since it is non-existent, has no beneficial effect; that the *violent effects* observed in patients under public treatment are due to contact, to the excitement of the imagination, and to *mechanical imitation* which involuntarily impels us to repeat that which strikes our senses. At the same time they are compelled to add, since it is an important observation, that the contact and repeated excitement of the imagination which produce the crises may become hurtful; that the spectacle of these crises is likewise dangerous *on account of the imitative faculty* which is a law of nature, and consequently that all treatment in public in which magnetism is employed must, in the end, be productive of evil results.

(Signed)   " B. FRANKLIN,

" MAJAULT,

" BAILLY,

" LEROY,

" D'ARCET,

" DeBORY,

" GUILLOTIN,

" LAVOISIER."

Shortly after this report was presented, the Royal Society of Medicine filed their report, in which they came to the same conclusions, one member, Laurent de Jussieu, dissenting, however. De Jussieu filed a separate report, in which he foreshadowed several points now universally acknowledged to be established truths. He declared that the experiments demonstrated the fact that man was capable of producing a sensible impression on his fellows through the agency of friction or contact. Charcot has shown that " the efficacy of contact and friction is proved by the existence in certain subjects of hypnogenic zones, of which the slightest stimulation produces somnambulism; that the irritation of hysteriogenic zones produces convulsions, and that these zones are generally seated in the hypochondriac or in the ovarian regions, on which Mesmer preferred to exercise his manipulations."

M. de Puységur, of Buzancy, near Soissons, gave, in 1784, the first account of hypnotism produced by manipulation, and the sequent phenomenon of healing by suggestion. He discovered that a patient whom he was treating for inflammation of the lungs, was thrown into a condition resembling sleep, yet retained consciousness, spoke aloud, and attended to his every-day affairs. De Puységur dis-

covered that, by suggestion, he could change
the current of this patient's thoughts and
make him do his bidding, at one moment
weeping as if in great sorrow, the next laugh-
ing as if convulsed with joy. "In his *waking
state* he was *simple* and *foolish*, but during the
crisis his intelligence was *remarkable.*" From
1784 to 1882 the science of hypnotism and the
treatment by suggestion was undergoing a
slow evolution, which finally culminated in
the work of M. Charcot, who at last took this
beneficial therapeutic agent from the hands of
charlatans and quacks, and placed it where it
belongs—among the remedial agents of repu-
table, scientific physicians. I have shown in
this brief *résumé* of the history of hypnotism
that certain classes of individuals were more
susceptible to this influence than others, and
that gender was a great and favorable factor.
The words previously italicized show that
women more frequently than men were influenced by hypnotic suggestion, and that these
favorable subjects always gave evidences of

hysteria or kindred neurotic lesions. The observations of Charcot and his pupils substantiate the experiences of the older scientists in this respect, and my own experience tallies with that of Charcot. I, therefore, deem it safe to advance the proposition, that the individuals who yield to the influence of hypnotism are always those who are neuropathic; Prof. Charcot wrote me, a short while before his death, that "he had come to the conclusion that all hypnotic subjects were the victims of neurotic lesion in some form or other." When we come to study the psychological phenomena accompanying hynoptism, we at once discover that this is a perfectly natural and absolutely truthful conclusion.

Man possesses two kinds of consciousness—an active, vigilant, co-ordinating consciousness, and a passive, pseudo-dormant, and, to a certain extent, incoherent and non-co-ordinating consciousness. We can readily prove the truth of this by observing certain phenomena which are to be noticed daily among ourselves. A

man falls into a "brown study," and, if gently
approached without being startled, he may be
asked questions which he will answer without
any conscious act on his part. His sub-consciousness, for the time being, holds him
beneath its sway; his active consciousness is
not so much obtunded but that he can answer
questions. Again, if a musician seated at a
piano and improvising, be approached and
gently questioned, he will answer the question
without ever ceasing his improvisation. Furthermore, the musician will play the most
difficult compositions while conversing. This
latter is due to automatism, a function of the
subliminal or *subconscious consciousness*. His
subconsciousness is elaborating the sweetest
harmonies, while his active consciousness, too,
is engaged in coherent and co-ordinating ideation.

Again, when the active consciousness is
stilled in slumber, subconsciousness sometimes
remains awake and makes itself evident in
dreams. The lack of rational thought-co-

ordination in subconsciousness is shown by the
greater or less extravagance and incoherence
of dreams. Everything, no matter how unnatural and extravagant, occurring to the
dreamer, is accepted by him as being natural
and consistent. When, however, his active
consciousness is aroused, he at once recognizes
the incoherence of his dreams. I hold, emphatically, that all dreams, when closely
studied, will show extravagance and incoherence. A dream may seem, at first, to be
entirely coherent, but, if the remembrance of
the dream be perfect and it be closely studied,
numerous incoherences will always be discovered.

We know how easy it is for us to lose ourselves in abstraction. We will sit for several
moments seemingly in profound thought, yet
when suddenly aroused and asked what engaged our thoughts, we are unable to tell.
We have been in a subconscious state, probably
reveling in the wildest vagaries. Fortunately
for us, degeneration has left no weakened spot

in our active consciousness on which to engraft the erotic imaginings of our incoherent sub-consciousness, consequently our waking moments of subconscious cerebration are blanks to our active, vigilant consciousness.

The favorable hypnotic subject, weakened by degeneration of some kind or other, is easily thrown into the subconscious state. The sudden entrance of a bright light into a darkened room; a loud noise; a sudden stillness after a prolonged noise; a breath of cold or warm air; the crackling of a lighted match, is all that is necessary, sometimes, to bring about hypnosis. I regard hypnosis as a state analogous to that of the "brown study" in which active consciousness is obtunded or asleep. It is, however, an intensified and aggravated form of mental abstraction, in which active consciousness is, more or less, profoundly affected. Why is it, that in the case of the favorable subject of hypnotism, the active consciousness can be so easily overcome? Simply because it is weakened by neurotic degeneration. That portion of the psychic system in which dwells active consciousness is always the first to degenerate and lose its tonicity. This is shown by the thousands of erotic mental habitudes and perversions that are to be noticed in neuropathic and psychopathic individuals. Active consciousness—the balance-wheel of the psychic system, becomes disordered and at once a flood of erotic fancies make themselves evident. It stands to reason that, in an individual, who shows by his actions and his thoughts that he is the victim of nervous degeneration, his active consciousness would be easily obtunded and put to sleep. This is, emphatically, the case, a fact that is clearly demonstrated by the favorable hypnotic subject, who is always neuropathic.

We know that subconsciousness is capable of receiving an impression and acting entirely independent of active consciousness—witness the phenomena of somnambulism.

When this fact is admitted the phenomena of hypnotic suggestion are readily accounted
9

for and understood. We have seen that many subjects fall into the hypnotic state when excited by the most trivial extraneous influences, such as the scratching of a match, a sudden noise, or a sudden stillness coming after long and continuous noise. Again, hypnosis can be produced by the favorable subject, sometimes, without the aid of extraneous influences. A patient of mine, an hysterical woman, would seat herself in a chair, "look cross-eyed," and, in a very few moments, become hypnotized. On one occasion, in order to test her condition, I commanded her to repeat the following lines, in lieu of the usual blessing, the next morning at breakfast : "*Juro tibi sanctæ per mystica sacra Dianæ me tibi venturam comitem sponsamque futuram.*" I wrote these lines on a slip of paper and gave it to her husband, a good Latin scholar, who declared that she repeated them word for word, giving the correct pronunciation, adding, however, the word "amen." This lady had never studied Latin and was not familiar with

the quotation.   Another patient, a young girl
who was psychopathic and neurasthenic, could
hypnotize herself by gazing at the brass ring
of a window curtain.   She and I discovered
this fact accidentally, I, having come upon her,
on one occasion, when she was in a hypnotized
state, intently gazing at the brass ring just
mentioned.   Repeated trials convinced me
that this girl could hypnotize herself at will
by gazing at the ring.   By a systematic course
of fasting and mental abstraction, thus weakening psychic vitality, the *tchogis* and *fakeers*
of India are enabled to throw themselves into
a hypnotic condition at will.   I have seen so-
called spirit-mediums and clairvoyants who
could bring about hypnosis a dozen times
daily if necessary.   Surely no one will assert
that these subjects are influenced by magnetism emanating from themselves or from outside objects.   One might just as well accept
the doctrines of Paracelsus and his disciples
of the sixteenth and seventeenth centuries!

   In conclusion let me state, that I am confident that hypnosis can be produced in the *favorable* subject, through many different avenues or agencies, and that every one of these agencies will be absolutely devoid of magnetism or any occult force!

VIRAGINITY AND EFFEMINATION.

In following up the chain of evolution in animal life from its inception in primordial protoplasm to its end, as we now find it, we discover that the interlinking organisms are, in the beginning, either. asexual or hermaphroditic. The moneron, the lowest form of animal life, simply multiplies by division. The different elements through which propagation and generation are carried on, are undoubtedly present even in the moneron, but are not differentiated. The moneron is an organless, structureless organism, consequently asexual. The cell, on the contrary, is hermaphroditic, for it contains within itself the necessary elements for reproducing itself. The amœba is the connecting link which connects all terrene life with primitive bathybian protoplasm, and is, strictly speaking, a true hermaphrodite. Ascending at once to the sixth stage in the ancestry of man, we come to the *acœlomi*, or

worms without body cavity. These worms
are phylogenetic, consequently hermaphroditic. I do not mean to say that these worms
have the organs of each sex equally developed; therefore, in the use of the word hermaphrodite, I use it in its broadest sense. I
simply mean that they are autogenetic. In
the *rhabdocœla* the sexual organs appear in
their simplest forms—a testis anterior to a
single or double ovary. Other gliding worms
have a more complex arrangement of the
sexual organs, but most of them are true
hermaphrodites. Next in the chain of evolutionary development, and one step nearer
man, we find the soft worms (*scolecidœ*); from
a branch of this family the parent group of
vertebrates was developed. The immediate
ancestor of the vertebrates was either the amphioxus (lancelet) or some other notochordate
animal, whose type is now extinct. Thus we
have traced hermaphroditism from the amœba
to the amphioxus, from the ancestor of the
parent cell to the ancestor of the vertebrates.

We could carry it further, but it is unnecessary. Effemination and viraginity are due directly to the influence of that strange law laid down by Darwin—the law of reversion to ancestral types. It is an effort of nature to return man to the old hermaphroditic form from which he was evolved. It is an effort on the part of nature to incorporate the individualities of the male and female, both physical and psychical, in one body. The phenomenon of atavism is more apt to occur in feeble types than in strong, healthy and well-developed types. Microcephalism, occurring, as it most frequently does, among ignorant, ill-nourished, and unhealthy people, is an example. Dolichocephalism and a flattening of the cranial arch, with corresponding loss of capacity in the skull—types that we see everywhere among the depraved and vicious—are other examples of this tendency of atavism to seize on weakened and unhealthy subjects. Effemination finds more victims among the wealthy and the educated than among the poor and uneducated. This phenomenon is a psychic rather than a physical hermaphroditism, and is directly traceable to the enervation produced by the habits of the wealthy and unemployed. Wealth begets luxury, luxury begets debauchery and consequent enervation. Periods of moral decadence in the life of a nation are always coincident with periods of luxury and great wealth, with consequent enervation and effemination; examples of this may be found in the histories of Rome, Greece, and France. During the reign of Louis XV., examples of effemination crowded into the court and vied with the royal fop in the splendor of their raiment and effeminacy of their bearing. Psychic hermaphroditism does not occur *naturally* in uncivilized or half-civilized races. The reason for this is patent. Atavism finds among them no weakened and enervated subjects on whom to perpetrate this strange travesty on nature.

Large cities are the hotbeds and breeding-places of the various neuroses. There

general paresis treads closely upon the heels
of sexual neurasthenia, while the victims of
hysteria and kindred ills are almost countless in their number. What wonder, then,
that the offspring of such parents should
be weak and neurasthenic, and fall easy victims to the thousand and one erotic fancies
which beset them! What wonder that here
atavism finds its richest field, and plays its
strangest and most fearful pranks, sending
men into the world with the tastes, desires,
and habits of women, and women with all the
mental habitudes of men! Juvenal wrote in
scathing, searing sarcasm of the degeneracy
of the Roman youth; effemination was very
prevalent, and this bitter satirist wrote burn-
ing words against their degrading and bestial
practices. It seems to me that we are beginning to need a Juvenal for this day and generation!

People divide themselves into classes, and
these classes are generally exceedingly clan-
nish. It is not considered " good form " to

marry out of the class to which an individual may belong, consequently, no new types of individuals are added. Luxury and debauchery enervate the classes which indulge in them. The people of these classes intermarry among themselves, no new blood is added, hence, in a very few generations, degeneration sets in.

Effemination and viraginity are common types of degeneration which always follow in the wake of luxury and debauchery. Effemination makes its appearance early in life. The young boy likes the society of girls; he plays with dolls, and, if permitted, will don female attire and dress his hair like a girl. He learns to sew, to knit, to embroider, to do "tatting." He becomes a connoisseur in female dress, and likes to discuss matters pertaining to the toilet of females. He does not care for boyish sports, and when he grows older, takes no pleasure in the amusements and pursuits of his masculine acquaintances. He prefers to spend his time with women and to engage in their employments and amusements. As the change in his psychic being becomes more pronounced and more overpowering, he will endeavor to approach the female in gait, attitude, and style of dress.

I have seen mothers guilty of incalculable harm by fostering such inclinations in their sons. They think (the thought is a natural one) that such perversions of taste indicate gentleness and kindliness, and induce their sons to continue in the practice of them, thus assisting atavism in its baneful work.

Effemination is a disease which, taken at its inception, can generally be eradicated and cured. As soon as it is discovered, the boy's surroundings should be changed; his mind should be directed into new channels, and his dormant boy's nature aroused. Outdoor exercise and a free intercourse with companions of his own sex should be made important factors in the treatment of an incipient effeminant. He should be carefully watched until *vita sexualis* has been established; he should then be taught the dangers of youthful follies and indiscretions.

A dandified man is always ridiculous, but when he adds to his foppery effemination, he then becomes contemptible.

Several years ago I had the opportunity of studying a pronounced effeminant. He is one of the best known young men of a Southern city, and is a leader in society. He took me to his "boudoir" and showed me his "lingerie." The words quoted are his own. His nightgowns were marvels of artistic needlework, as far as I was able to judge, and were made by himself. His nightcaps were "sweetly pretty," and one of them was a "perfect dream of beauty." On his dressing-table were all the accessories of a modern society woman's toilet, including rouge, powder, a complete manicure set, and numerous bottles of perfumes and toilet waters. In his wardrobe he had, displayed on forms, some six or eight corsets and chemisettes—"corset-covers," as he designated them.

This man's voice and manner of speaking are decidedly feminine; all the little mannerisms and affectations of a society woman being faithfully reproduced. I understand from his associates that he is a splendid business man, and that not a breath of scandal has ever tarnished his good name. He was reared by his mother, and never associated with boys until his sixteenth year. I understood from him that she always treated him as a girl, and consulted him in all things pertaining to her toilet. He seemed utterly unconscious of his anomalous condition, and as his business associates are gentlemen, and his intimate friends are ladies, he may drift through life without a single jar to mar the serenity of his existence.

Viraginity is, comparatively, an infrequent occurrence, but under its influence the unfortunate victims are guilty of startling vagaries. The recent case of Alice Mitchell, who killed Miss Ward, at Memphis, Tenn., is an example of pronounced viraginity. We see daily in the newspapers accounts of women who masquerade as men, and history abounds in like

instances. The celebrated writer Count Sandor V. was a woman who posed as a man,
and who was in fact Sarolta (Charlotte),
Countess V. "Among many foolish things
that her father encouraged in her was the fact
that he brought her up as a boy, called her
Sandor, allowed her to ride, drive, and hunt,
admiring her muscular energy." At the age
of thirteen she ran away from school, where
she had been sent by her mother, and returned
home. " Sarolta returned to her mother, who,
however, could do nothing and was compelled
to allow her daughter to again become Sandor,
wear male clothes, and, at least once a year, to
fall in love with persons of her own sex."

Mothers, early in life, though not from any
sense of danger to their daughters, begin to
eradicate the tom-boy inclinations in their
female children ; hence the comparative infre-
quency of viraginity. The congenital viragint
will always remain somewhat masculine in her
tastes and ideas, but her inclinations and
desires having been turned toward femininity

early in life, she will escape the horrors of
complete viraginity or gynandry. The vic‑
tim of effemination, however, is saved by no
such accidental forethought. The ignorant
mother fosters feminine inclinations and
desires in her effeminate son until his psychic
being becomes entirely changed, and not even
the establishment of *vita sexualis* will save him
from effemination.

An only son, who is in the least degree
neurasthenic, runs the risk of becoming an
effeminant under the tutelage of a loving but
ignorant mother who encourages his feminine
tastes and inclinations. A young man of
my acquaintance, who is an only son, is so
situated. This young man devotes his entire
attention to matters of the toilet. He paints
his cheeks and powders his face; even his
eyebrows and eyelashes are anointed with
some dark-colored ointment or pomade.

Effemination and viraginity are more prevalent in the Old World than in the United
States. The civilization and settlement of the

United States are, comparatively speaking, new. The people are, as yet, a young, strong, and vigorous nation. Years of luxury and debauchery have not yet brought the penalty of enervation and neurasthenia to the *masses*, though, in certain circles of society, it is becoming painfully evident that that penalty is being even now exacted.

In this article I have described only mild types of viraginity and effemination. In the more pronounced types of these singular examples of atavism or reversion, the victims commit the most unheard of and the most unnatural acts.

Almost every case of effemination or viraginity can be cured if recognized and treated in its incipiency. The parents should be the physicians. They should keep a watchful supervision over their offspring, and as soon as any evidences of effemination or viraginity become apparent, treatment, both physical and psychical, should at once be instituted.

Effemination has occasioned the downfall of

many nations; let us guard against it with all our power. Let us train up our boys to be manly men, and our girls to be womanly women.

BORDERLANDS AND CRANKDOM.

When that bilious critic and merciless crucifier of human foibles, Carlyle, himself a degenerate, wrote that nine tenths of the world were fools, he was much nearer truth than most men think. When we take an introspective view of our sane personality, we shudder to see how near it is to the borderlands of insanity and the bizarre and eccentric world of crankdom. There hardly lives a man who does not possess some eccentricity, or who does not cherish, hidden, perhaps, deep within himself, some small delusion, which he is ashamed to acknowledge to the outside world. Social relations and the iron rules of custom hold in place the balance-wheel of many a disordered mind. The mental equipoise is kept at the normal standard only by the powerful aid of the will, supported and assisted by extraneous adjuvants, such as fear of punishment, fear of personal harm, and, above all, by the fear of ridicule. Many a man hugs his delusions closely to his heart, indulges them only in the secret recesses of his soul, and, their sole owner and acquaintance, carries them with him to his grave.

Any man who has a retentive memory, and one capable of minute analysis, can look back in his life and recall moments when his insane personality got the better of his will, and ran riot in forbidden pathways. He may not have committed an insane act; yet the thought, the impulse, the delusion was there and only outside influences kept it from breaking forth. Who fails to remember certain times in his life when he has had an almost overpowering desire to cry out in church, or to laugh on some sad or solemn occasion; or, having a razor in his hand, has had an impulse, sudden and intense, to draw it across his throat; or, being on some high place, has been seized with the desire to hurl himself downward? This shows how near indeed the healthy mind ever hovers on the borderlands of insanity.

Man stands so close to the portals of insanity that he can look through the gateway, when he takes an introspective view of his psychical being, and can see the phantoms and mental ghosts of his insane personality.

We have every reason to believe that, among civilized races, there is a vast amount of latent insanity. Taking the tables of our insane asylums, we find a thousand and one causes given as the exciting factors in the mental overthrow. Love, religion, anger, disappointment, etc., down through the long list of psychic and æsthetic emotions, until it seems as though even a breath of wind would be sufficient to destroy the mental equipoise.

Among savage and uncivilized races, insanity is of infrequent occurrence. Only when a race begins to elevate itself and take on a higher view of morality, when new rules and new laws, new customs and innovations, tending to place individuals in a state of comparison, arise, does insanity make its appearance. The untutored savage, living in a state of communism, is untroubled by the jealousies and heart-burnings of his civilized congener. He lives in the to-day and allows the to-morrow to care of itself. Devoid of ambition, a mere animal, sensual and indolent, he cares only for the gratification of his physical desires. The mental attributes of a civilized being are, in him, wanting.

Psychos is the result of evolutionary development, and the chief reason why insanity is not as prevalent in the savage as in the civilized man, is because the brain of the savage lacks development. I do not wish to convey the idea that insanity is purely psychical in its nature. Insanity is the result of a material change in the structure of the brain produced by morbific action. The manifestations of insanity are merely the symptoms of a disease that involves the brain. The savage has less development of psychical function, consequently he is less liable to mental lesion. I mean by psychical function that portion of

the brain in which psychos has its origin.
Alienists consider the habits of men as being
the factor in the production of insanity. Habits and heredity are undoubted factors in the
production of diseased minds, and, in fact, are
the chief agents. You can not, however, expect to find a disordered function where that
function is absent. Savages have paresis,
apoplexy, and imbecility, seldom or never insanity. The reason is patent—they lack the
psychic function, that peculiar element, whatever it may be, which raises civilized man so
high above them. That this element can be
developed in savages I do not for one instant
deny. The ploughshare of evolutionary civilization will bring it to the surface sooner or
later, and when it does insanity follows. I
have only to point to the American negro to
prove the truth of my proposition; even he is
partially exempt, simply because his civilization is of such recent date that his brain has
not yet acquired its full quota of the psychic
element.

I will venture to assert, so true is the fact that insanity is the product of civilization, that, if it were not for the combating influences of social laws, assisted not a little by scientific medical aid, all North America could not contain the vast and enormous army that would constitute the civilized world's array of lunatics.

There seems to be in the minds of men an instinctive awe of anything that appertains to the insane. In olden times a disordered mind was considered of divine or diabolic origin as it evinced good or evil tendencies. This belief lasted even until the present century. Many old women who were the victims of senile dementia and kindred ills, were accused of witchcraft and intercourse with the devil, here in the United States, not a century ago. Witches were executed in England and men burned at the stake in Spain, not two hundred years ago, for the crime of demoniacal possession. Even in this enlightened age men are accustomed to consider in-

sanity rather from its psychical standpoint
than from its physical aspect. They do not
take into consideration the fact that insanity
is due to a physical lesion, and that its vagaries are but the symptoms of brain disease or
brain deformity. The inhabitants of the borderlands are invested with a certain shadowy
mystery which separates them from the rest
of mankind, and which makes them appear to
us as denizens of another psychical world than
ours.

In the Middle Ages, cranks, whose eccentricities took a religious turn, were considered holy. St. Simon Stylites was a very
pronounced crank, and a very holy man also,
because he chose to live the greater portion
of his life perched on a pillar seventy feet high.
St. Anthony was another holy crank who
never, in all his life, washed his feet. Poor
Joan of Arc was burned at the stake because
she was "possessed of a false and lying devil."
She has been recently canonized by the same
church that burned her, and thus, in a meas-

ure, had justice done her. I do not think, however, that this is any recompense for the terrible agony inflicted on this unfortunate victim of hystero-epilepsy.

Says Maudsley in "Responsibility in Mental Disease": "Some of the prophets of the Old Testament presented symptoms which can hardly be interpreted as other than the effects of madness; certainly if they were not mad, they imitated very closely some of its most striking features." Jeremiah takes a long journey to the river Euphrates and hides a linen girdle in a hole of a rock. He then returns home and in a few days makes the same journey, and finds the girdle rotten and good for nothing. Ezekiel digs a hole in the wall of his house, and through it removes his household goods, instead of through the door. Hosea marries a prostitute because he said he had been commanded by God so to do. Isaiah stripped himself naked and paraded up and down in the sight of all the people.

Some of the greatest changes in the world's

history have been effected by dwellers in the borderlands. Mahomet was an epileptic, and his first vision was the result of an epileptic convulsion or seizure. The character of his visions was exactly like that of those visions which an epileptic sees and describes at the present time. Mahomet believed in his visions, and, what is more, got more than half the world to believe in them also. Gautama was a dweller in the borderlands, yet his followers now number five hundred millions.

The novel mode in which an insane man regards things may be an inspiration which reflection could never attain, and it sometimes happens that opinions which seem to the world to be the ravings of a madman, have turned out to be true. The insane man has the world against him, and though he may pose for a short time as a reformer, sooner or later lands in the asylum.

It sometimes happens that the crank will succeed in getting converts. A notable instance is Schweinfurth, or "the Christ," as he

calls himself. I am firmly convinced that this
man believes in his delusions. One thing is
certain, and that is, his disciples believe in him
implicitly. This man is dangerous to society,
inasmuch as he has caused the separation of
several wives from their husbands; the wives
abandoning their husbands to follow him to
" Heaven," as he calls his farm house.

The crank is, generally, a harmless individual, and is not anti-social unless his delusions
take the form of homicidal impulse, pyroma-
nia, kleptomania, etc.

Homicidal impulse is the most dangerous
to society of the many mental vagaries and
derangements which afflict the dwellers in
the borderlands. Its invasion is sudden and
its impulse is, generally, overpowering. A
man may be walking the streets presumably
in perfect health, and yet have, all the while,
a voice whispering in his ear " kill, kill." His
insane desire at length reaches its acme, and
he throws aside every mental restraint and
kills the first individual he may chance to

meet. Again, he may desire to kill some particular individual, and will carefully and systematically arrange his plans for the successful enactment of the homicide. The murderers of Garfield and Harrison probably belong to this latter class, though in the case of Prendergast, the slayer of Mayor Harrison, this opinion may be erroneous. There is something about his photograph that leads me to believe that he is a moral imbecile, rather than an intellectual dyscrasiac.

A clerk in a solicitor's office, at Alton, Hampshire, England, one afternoon took a walk outside the town, when he met some children. He persuaded one of these, a girl of nine, to go with him into a neighboring garden. A short while after, he was seen walking quietly home; he was seen to wash himself in the river and then go back to his office. The little girl did not return home, and, search having been instituted, her dismembered body was found strewn about the garden. The clerk was arrested, and in his diary was found this entry, recently made : "Killed a little girl; it was fine and hot." This man was either a sadistic sexual pervert, or a victim of homicidal impulse. Maudsley gives this instance as an example of the latter, while Kraft-Ebing gives it as an example of the former. There is a great difference between these two mental derangements. The victim of homicidal impulse kills without any ulterior object, while the sadist kills in order to gratify his unnatural and perverted sexual appetite.

The victim of homicidal impulse is, to all outward appearances, perfectly sane otherwise. His impulse frequently leaves him for years and then returns with overpowering force.

Epileptics who have just passed through violent convulsions, will frequently attack bystanders with great fury. Some alienists declare that homicidal mania is frequently only a masked epilepsy. All epileptics should be carefully watched; they may become dangerous to society at any moment. Numerous instances are recorded of murder committed by sufferers from *petit mal,* a form of epilepsy. I once saw a negro walk up to a white man, who was a stranger and unknown by him, and fell him to the earth by striking him with a club. The negro was arrested, and the next day swore that he was entirely unconscious of having struck anyone. It was proven on his trial that he was subject to mild epileptic attacks.

I believe that all suicides are due to mental aberration. It may be the result of a momentary and sudden loss of mental equipoise, or the final and fatal ending of a premeditated desire carried through days, weeks, months, and even years.

We see a man, blessed with everything that makes life enjoyable, genial, gay, with a ready smile and kindly word for everyone, suddenly, in a moment, pass forever out into the unknown—self-killed, a victim of his own creation. We stand amazed! Why did he do it? We can find nothing in his past or present condition to warrant such an action.

He was the victim of momentary aberration, or, perhaps, deep in his mind, buried and hidden even from himself, there dwelt a desire for self-slaughter, when a "physical pain, an unexpected impression, a moral affection, an indiscreet proposition" uncovered this desire, and he at once committed the deed!

There are epidemics of suicide. Let the papers chronicle some peculiar method of suicide selected by some unfortunate, and others will immediately follow his example. Unconscious cerebration also hurls many souls out of the world. I was called to see a gentleman who had attempted suicide by slashing the radial artery at the wrist. I found him holding a compress on the severed vessel and greatly alarmed. He swore to me that he was totally unconscious how he had come to do the deed, and that he did not know that he had cut himself until he felt the pain and saw the blood flowing from the wound!

Viraginity and effemination, while not mental insanities, strictly speaking, are, nevertheless, mental deformities, and their unfortunate victims are dwellers in the borderlands. Mild forms of these types of degeneration are very abundant. The effeminate, cigarette-smoking, soda-drinking young man of the comic weeklies, and the loud, horsy, slang-using, vulgar, masculine young woman are seen everywhere.

Effemination and viraginity are the results of the weakening effects of luxury and consequent debauchery. Nations, time and again, have felt the dire effects of effemination and have sunk beneath them. The Grecian, the Roman, and the Egyptian nations are familiar examples. The satirists of the golden age of the Latin people dipped their *stili*, metaphorically, in gall and bitter wormwood and berated the effeminate nobility time and again. One of them advised the Roman ladies to look for *men* among the gladiators and the peasants! Anacreon's poems are filled with allusions to effemination and the delights of psychic hermaphroditism.

In the time of Louis XIV., of France, the royal palaces were filled to repletion with effeminants, who vied with the women in the splendor of their robes and the salacious eccentricities of their conduct. The case of Alice Mitchell, who killed Freda Ward in Memphis not long ago, was one of pronounced viraginity.

Fortunately, for the good of the community at large, there are, comparatively speaking, few viragints. The careful mother restrains, tempers, and abolishes the hoydenish habits of her "tom-boy" girl early in life, and turns her thoughts toward feminine pursuits and desires. The unfortunate effeminant, however, is encouraged in his feminine tastes and habits by his unwise mother, who likes her boy to sit beside her and sew and knit, if he so desires. She discusses matters of the toilet with him, and, in fact, treats him as she would a daughter. In the end, his psychic

11

hermaphroditism becomes complete, and one more unfortunate goes out into the world to swell the ranks of crankdom!

Kleptomaniacs are greatly to be pitied, for they are generally women in whom the moral sense is very much developed. The victim of kleptomania will steal any and everything; they are like magpies in this respect. An acquaintance of mine, a most estimable lady, a devout Christian, and a most exemplary wife and mother, is the most incorrigible thief I ever saw. She has often picked my pockets while I was engaged about her sick-bed. The merchants of the city where she lives know her infirmity, watch her while she is in their shops, and respectfully and kindly relieve her of her pilferings when she starts to leave. She expresses great sorrow for her unfortunate insane impulse, and has often begged her husband to have her placed in an asylum. This he refuses to do, as she is perfectly sane otherwise. The husband was called away for several weeks, and, on his return, took me to his house

and showed me her room. In the room were
the objects stolen during his absence. It was
the most miscellaneous collection of valuables
and trash I ever saw. She had gathered together everything from a darning-needle to a
tombstone, a small specimen of the latter forming a unit of this heterogeneous whole. This
form of mental dyscrasia is much more frequent than people suppose, and the antece-
dents of shop-lifters and the like should be
carefully examined before a judgment on their
criminality is passed.

"Eccentricity is certainly not always insanity, but there can be no question that it is
often the outcome of insane temperament, and
may approach very near to, or actually pass
into, insanity." Alienists rely on the eccentric
and peculiar changes which take place in the
characters of their patients, who either present
themselves or are brought to them for treatment, to establish their diagnosis. If a mod-
est and truthful man suddenly becomes a
braggart and a liar; or, if a humane man

becomes cruel, or a neat man slovenly, there
is reason to suspect brain trouble.   The intel-
lect may appear intact, so also the reasoning
powers, but these eccentricities indicate a
deviation which may lead to mental destruction.   The last faculty to develop in the mind
of man is the moral faculty; this faculty is
the one first lost by diseased brains.   If a
man, who suddenly becomes dissolute and
licentious (who, heretofore, has led a virtuous,
moral life), be examined, in nine cases in ten
his brain will be found to be diseased.   The
little cloud, which at first is no larger than a
man's hand, grows ever larger and larger, and
in the end overspreads the entire mental sky!

THE METHODS OF THE RIOTING STRIKER AN EVIDENCE OF DEGENERATION.

The doctrines of communism, socialism, and nihilism are essentially atavistic doctrines, inasmuch as they revert to a state of society existing thousands and thousands of years ago, when all mankind were savages. It is only by a study of primitive folk as we find them to-day that we are enabled to form any idea of our own status before civilization raised us to our present elevated position. It will hardly be necessary, in order to demonstrate this proposition, to cite more than one instance of communism as we now find it existing in a primitive race of people, though many such could be cited. Therefore I will call attention only to a single tribe of communists, the Aleutians,* living on our own continent. It

---

(*) Throughout this book I speak of the Aleutians as they *were* when first discovered, and not as they are now. Their customs have been considerably modified by their association with civilization.

is a mistaken idea to suppose that, in the inception of his history, man was isolated and lived apart from his fellow-beings; that "the first individual reproduced himself in male and female, and of this couple, created superb and vigorous, intelligent and beautiful, was born the first family, which expanded into a tribe, then into peoples and nations." This was a theory taught years ago, before paleontology became a science and taught us otherwise. Our pithecoid ancestors began with a communal life, and, instead of the individual being the father of the society, the society has been the father of the individual. Says Reclus:

"Communal was the habitation, and communal the wives with their children; the men pursued the same prey, and devoured it together after the manner of wolves; all felt, thought, and acted in concert. Everything leads us to believe that at the outset collectivism was at its maximum and individualism at its minimum. The communal dwelling appears to us to have been the support of the collective life, and the great medium of the earliest civilization."

In the *kachims* of the Aleutians we see the autotypes of the communal dwelling-places of *our* savage ancestors; likewise their customs and their beliefs have their archetypes in the political and social economics of *our* primitive forebears. It is to some such state of savage irresponsibility that the doctrines of Bellamy and his followers would hurry us in the end, if they were carried out to their full extent. Man would have to lose, necessarily, that individuality and responsibility which he has acquired through thousands of years of inherited experiences. Could he do this, man might attain to the Utopia described by Bellamy, and become the autotype of the ant and the bee and others of the social hymenoptera. But he can never do it without losing that which makes him so immeasurably superior to the savage—his civilization. Civilization, in its purity, demands an individualism totally inconsistent with the tenets and doctrines of communism and socialism. The innate *ego* of civilized man is too self-assertive to allow him to banish it for any length of time, and, as his psychical development is always on the increase, it will ever be growing stronger and stronger.

The surroundings demanding the communistic customs of our savage ancestors no longer exist, and a belief in any such doctrine at the present time is unquestionably an instance of psychical atavism. Fortunately for civilization, the majority of mankind are not degenerate; therefore these atavistic tendencies of the minority are held in check. Every now and then, however, the degenerate element bursts through the restraining bonds of social laws and customs, and makes its savage nature apparent in the strike or the boycott, accompanied, as they always are, by riots and lawlessness.

Any man has the right to stop work whenever he wishes, if he is not under contract and

can legally do so, but no man has a right to
stop another man from working if he so desires.
Such an act would be clearly anti-social, therefore criminal. It is here that the strike shows
that it is the offspring of degeneration, for the
strikes of to-day are invariably accompanied
by anti-social acts that at once place them
among the *instrumenta belli* of the savage.
Arson, murder, and theft belong to the cardi-
nal virtues according to the tenets laid down
by savages and moral imbeciles, and arson,
murder, and theft invariably march in the
van of the strike.

Communism or socialism must necessarily
form a factor in any movement of labor
against capital. This fact is always bitterly
denied by the more conservative and politic
of the labor leaders, yet the active strikers
who engage personally in the strike unhesi-
tatingly assert that their main object is to
place themselves more nearly on a par with
their wealthy employers. Now, having shown
that communism is an atavistic doctrine, and

that the strike invariably carries with it an
element of communism, and is therefore necessarily atavistic, let us examine into the causes
which produce this strange desire to revert
to the customs, habits, and beliefs of our barbarous progenitors.

The causes of degeneration are manifold,
and can not be enumerated in a paper like
this. Suffice it to say that insufficient food, in-
temperance, and a disregard for the bars of con-
sanguinity in marital relations are some of the
prime factors in the production of degenerate
beings. I have shown elsewhere that degeneration is the cause of the various forms of
sexual perversion with which civilized man
is afflicted (*vide* "Effemination and Viraginity"), and that it is likewise the main factor
in the production of a distinct type of abnormal man, the congenital criminal (*vide* New
York Medical Record, January, 1894 : *Criminal Anthropology*, and American Naturalist,
June, 1894 : *The Recidivist*). When we come
to examine the personnel of a striking mob,

we at once discover that it is made up, to
a great extent, of foreigners and the descendants of foreigners. And when we examine
each individual, we will discover that he differs
more or less from normal man, and that these
abnormalties in face and figure form a distinct
type. These abnormalties are the unmistakable signs of degeneration. Of course I
have reference to *the strike in which lawlessness
is evinced;* throughout this article I mean no
other.

The struggle for existence among the lower
classes of Europe has been exceedingly hard.
On account of the numerous wars which have
occurred during the last millenary period, the
burden of taxation has been very heavy, rents
have been very high, and the consequent
struggle of the laboring classes for a bare
existence has been very severe. Physical
development has been retarded, and even
turned back, and psychical atavism has made
its appearance. Both mind and body have
retrograded. Instead of advancing toward a

higher civilization, the peasantry of most of the European nations have dropped back.

The phenomenon of atavism occurs in feeble types, not in strong, healthy, well-developed types. Microcephalism, occurring, as it most frequently does, among ignorant, ill-nourished, and unhealthy people, is an example. Dolichocephalism, and a flattening of the cranial arch, with corresponding loss of capacity in the skull—types that we see everywhere among the individuals now being discussed, are other examples of this tendency of atavism to seize on weakened and unhealthy subjects.

Degeneration finds victims among the rich as well as among the poor, but among the wealthy the atavistic abnormalities are generally psycho-sexual in character.. The rich become effeminate, weak, and immoral, and the lower classes, taking advantage of this moral lassitude, and, led on by their savage inclinations, undertake strikes, mobs, boycotts, and riots. If it were not for the restraining influence of the sober, level-headed middle classes—the true police of the world—civilization would be swept from the face of the globe, and men would become savages like the communal tribes of the Aleutian Islands!

The native-born American working-man, descended from Anglo-Saxon ancestors, has not yet been attacked by degeneration. In this fruitful land his struggle for existence has been easy; consequently, his physical and psychical beings have not been held in check and turned back by the exigencies of his surroundings, but, on the contrary, have been greatly developed. He takes broad and elevated views of sociological questions. He recognizes the fact that each man is the architect of his own fortune, and that success depends on the intrinsic worth of each individual. In fact, he is the product of a higher civilization, which decrees that the individual, and not the commune, is the great desideratum. He knows that labor is a marketable commodity, and that it will always bring its

own price unless the market becomes overstocked.   And now we come to the key of
the whole situation.   The labor-market is, to
a certain extent, overstocked.

The country has become filled with laborers,
the vast majority of whom are degenerate foreigners, who are ready for any form of lawlessness and riot suggested by their essentially
anti-social natures.   A mere casual survey of
the various strikes which have occurred in the
United States during the last decade will show
that an overwhelming majority of the individuals constituting the strike are foreigners, and
descendants of foreigners.

It is true that there are native-born descendants of Anglo-Saxon ancestors in the ranks of
the strikers, but they are few in number, and
are uniformly led on by emotions and desires
founded on higher principles than those which
actuate their foreign associates.   These men
are amenable to reason, and do not commit acts
of lawlessness unless forced to do so by their
anarchistic fellow-strikers.   The fear of bodily

harm, or the fear of being considered a cow-
ard, have made many a law-abiding man a
criminal!

The psychical habitudes of a few of the individuals under discussion have been inherited
from ancestors who have always been of low
types, but the majority of them are *bona fide*
degenerates, made so by inheritance as well as
by their surroundings.

The Russian and Bohemian laborers who
immigrate to America are, and always have
been, semi-civilized, but the Italians, Germans, Huns, Poles, Frenchmen, and Austrians
who are to be found among rioting laborers,
are clearly a degenerate class of human beings.
The anthropologist can detect the physical
signs of degeneration in these people at a
glance. Their physical characteristics mark
them out at once to be abnormal types of the
human race, with such a striking family resemblance that individuals of entirely different
nationalities look alike. This same family
resemblance is to be found among congenital

criminals. In point of fact, the congenital criminal and the anarchist, both victims of degeneration, differ very little. The congenital criminal's anti-social acts are generally individual, while the anti-social acts of the communistic anarchist are communal or collective. Of the two individuals, I consider the communist by far the more dangerous to society.

In conclusion, let me say that I believe that the immigration laws are wholly to blame for the labor riots which agitate the country. Immigration is practically unrestricted, and year after year Europe pours into the United States multitudes of degenerate human beings, who, incited by the freedom of American institutions, and without the fear of summary punishment (such as would be meted out to them in the countries from whence they came), immediately give free rein to their atavistic imaginations, and, whenever they think that the favorable moment has arrived, plunge into anarchy and lawlessness. These

people are savages, and should not be treated
as civilized beings. They are not amenable to
those arguments which would undoubtedly
influence and prevail were they *normal* civilized men and women; consequently it is folly
to argue with them. Their ideas of social
economy are totally different from those of
normal civilized men, and the sooner the
world recognizes this fact the better will it be
for civilization.

When the Indians out West go on the war-
path we know how to control them. The
psychologist considers the anarchist as being
no higher, psychically, than the Indian!

12

GENIUS AND DEGENERATION.

That the psychical function or intellectuality is frequently developed at the expense of the physical organism is well known, and that genius is seldom or never unaccompanied by physical and mental degeneration is a fact that can be no longer denied. I use the word degeneration in its broadest sense, and intend it to include all kinds of abnormalities. The facts noted above are by no means recent knowledge, but were vaguely recognized and commented on centuries and decades of centuries ago by the Hebrews and kindred races of people. The Hebrew word *nabi* means either madman or prophet, and it is now admitted that most of the prophets gave evidences of insanity as well as genius. The Greeks and the Romans recognized this kinship, and we read in the Bible of a certain Festus, who, when confronted by a man of genius, and being unable to answer his arguments, said to him, " Paul, much learning hath made thee mad!" Lauvergne, when speaking of the oxycephalic (sugar-loaf) skull, an unquestionable example of degeneration, wrote many years ago, "This head announces the monstrous alliance of the most eminent faculty of man, genius, with the most pronounced impulses to rape, murder, and theft."

The purpose of this paper is to show that wherever genius is observed, we find it accompanied by degeneration, which is evinced by physical abnormalties or mental eccentricities. It is a strange fact, however, and one not noticed by Lombroso, or any other writer, as far as I know, that mechanical geniuses, or those who, for the most part, deal with material facts, do not, as a rule, show any signs of degeneration. I have only to instance Darwin, Galileo, Edison, Watts, Rumsey, Howe, and Morse to prove the truth of this assertion. It is only the genius of æstheticism, the genius of the emotion, that is generally accompanied by unmistakable signs of degeneration.

Saul, the first king of Israel, was a man of genius and, at times, a madman. We read that, before his coronation, he was seized with an attack of madness and joined a company of kindred eccentrics. His friends and acquaintances were naturally surprised and exclaimed: "Is Saul among the prophets?" *i. e.*, "Has Saul become insane?" Again, we are told that he was suddenly seized with an attack of homicidal impulse, and tried to kill David. Before this time he had had repeated attacks of madness, which only the harp of David could control and subdue. David himself was a man whose mental equilibrium was not well established, as his history clearly indicates. He forsook his God, indulged in licentious practices, and was, withal, a very immoral man at times. At his time, the Hebrews had reached a high degree of civilization. Abstract ethics had become very much developed, and any example of great immor-

ality occurring during this epoch is proof positive of atavism or degeneration.

As I have intimated before, many of the ancient Hebrew prophets, who were unquestionably men of genius, gave evidences of insanity ;
notably Jeremiah, who made a long journey to
the River Euphrates, where he hid a linen girdle. He returned home, and in a few days made
the same journey and found the girdle rotten
and good for nothing; Ezekiel, who dug a
hole in the wall of his house, through which
he removed his household goods, instead of
through the door; Hosea, who married a prostitute, because God, so he declared, had told
him so to do; and Isaiah, who stripped himself naked and paraded up and down in sight
of all the people. King Solomon, a man of
pre-eminent genius, was mentally unbalanced.
The " Song of Solomon" shows very clearly
that he was a victim of some psychical disorder, sexual in its character and origin. The
poems of Anacreon are lascivious, lustful, and

essentially carnal, and history informs us that he was a sexual pervert.

Swinburne's poems shows clearly the mental bias of their author, who is described as being peculiar and eccentric. Many of the men of genius who have assisted in making the history of the world have been the victims of epilepsy. Julius Cæsar, military leader, statesman, politician, and author, was an epileptic. Twice on the field of battle he was stricken down by this disorder. On one occasion, while seated at the tribune, he was unable to rise when the senators, consuls, and prætors paid him a visit of ceremony and honor. They were offended at his seeming lack of respect, and retired, showing signs of anger. Cæsar returned home, stripped off his clothes, and offered his throat to be cut by anyone. He then explained his conduct to the senate, saying that he was the victim of a malady which, at times, rendered him incapable of standing. During the attacks of this disorder " he felt shocks in his limbs, became giddy, and at last lost consciousness." Molière was the victim of epilepsy; so also was Petrarch, Flaubert, Charles V., Handel, St. Paul, Peter the Great, and Dostoieffsky; Paganini, Mozart, Schiller, Alfieri, Pascal, Richelieu, Newton, and Swift were the victims of diseases epileptoid in character.

Many men of genius have suffered from spasmodic and choreic movements, notably Lenau, Montesquieu, Buffon, Dr. Johnson, Santeuil, Crébillon, Lombardini, Thomas Campbell, Carducci, Napoleon, and Socrates.

Suicide, essentially a symptom of mental disorder, has hurried many a man of genius out into the unknown. The list begins with such eminent men as Zeno, Cleanthes, Dionysius, Lucan, and Stilpo, and contains the names of such immortals as Chatterton, Blount, Haydon, Clive, and David.

Alcoholism and morphinism, or an uncontrollable desire for alcohol or opium in some form or other, are now recognized as evidences of degeneration. Men of genius, both

in the Old World and in the New, have shown
this form of degeneration.   Says Lombroso:
"Alexander died after having emptied ten
times the goblet of Hercules, and it was, without doubt, in an alcoholic attack, while pursu-
ing naked the infamous Thais, that he killed
his dearest friend.   Cæsar was often carried
home intoxicated on the shoulders of his sol-
diers.   Neither Socrates, nor Seneca, nor
Alcibiades, nor Cato, nor Peter the Great
(nor his wife Catherine, nor his daughter
Elizabeth) were remarkable for their absti-
nence.   One recalls Horace's line, '*Narratur
et prisci Cantonis sæpe mero caluisse virtus.*'
Tiberius Nero was called by the Romans
Biberius Mero.   Septimius Severus and Mahomet II. succumbed to drunkenness or *deli-
rium tremens.*"

Among the men and women of genius of
the Old World who abused the use of alcohol
and opium, were Coleridge, James Thomson,
Carew, Sheridan, Steele, Addison, Hoffman,
Charles Lamb, Madame de Staël, Burns, Sav-

age, Alfred de Musset, Kleist, Caracci, Jan Steen, Morland Turner (the painter), Gérard de Nerval, Hartley Coleridge, Dussck, Handel, Glück, Praga, Rovani, and the poet Somerville. This list is by no means complete, as the well-informed reader may see at a glance; it serves to show, however, how very often this form of degeneration makes its appearance in men of genius.

In men of genius the moral sense is sometimes obtunded, if not altogether absent. Sallust, Seneca, and Bacon were suspected felons. Rousseau, Byron, Foscolo, and Caresa were grossly immoral, while Casanova, the gifted mathematician, was a common swindler. Murat, Rousseau, Clement, Didcrot, Praga, and Oscar Wilde were sexual perverts.

Genius, like insanity, lives in a world of its own, hence we find few, if any, evidences of human affection in men of genius. Says Lombroso: "I have been able to observe men of genius when they had scarce reached the age of puberty; they did not manifest the

deep aversions of moral insanity, but I have
noticed among all a strange apathy for everything which does not concern them; as
though, plunged in the hypnotic condition,
they did not perceive the troubles of others,
or even the most pressing needs of those who
were dearest to them; if they observed them,
they grew tender, at once hastening to attend
them; but it was a fire of straw, soon extin-
guished, and it gave place to indifference and
weariness."

This emotional anæsthesia is indicative of
psychical atavism, and is an unmistakable evidence of degeneration. Lombroso gives a
long list of the men of genius who were celi-
bates. I will mention a few of those with
whom the English-speaking world is most
familiar: Kant, Newton, Pitt, Fox, Beethoven,
Galileo, Descartes, Locke, Spinoza, Leibnitz,
Gray, Dalton, Hume, Gibbon, Macaulay,
Lamb, Bentham, Leonardo da Vinci, Coper-
nicus, Reynolds, Handel, Mendelssohn, Meyer-
beer, Schopenhauer, Camoëns, and Voltaire.

La Bruyère says of men of genius: "These men have neither ancestors nor descendants; they themselves form their entire posterity."

There is a form of mental obliquity which the French term *folie du doute*. It is characterized by an incertitude in thought coördination, and often leads its victims into the perpetration of nonsensical and useless acts. Men of genius are very frequently afflicted with this form of mental disorder. Dr. Johnson, who was a sufferer from *folie du doute*, had to touch every post he passed. If he missed one he had to retrace his steps and touch it. Again, if he started out of a door on the wrong foot he would return and make another attempt, starting out on the foot which he considered the correct one to use. Napoleon counted and added up the rows of windows in every street through which he passed. A celebrated statesman, who is a personal friend of the writer, can never bear to place his feet on a crack in the pavement or floor. When walking he will carefully step over and beyond all cracks or crevices. This idiosyncracy annoys him greatly, but the impulse is imperative, and he can not resist it.

Those who have been intimately associated with men of genius have noticed that they are very frequently amnesic or " absent-minded." Newton once tried to stuff his niece's finger into the bowl of his lighted pipe, and Rovelle would lecture on some subject for hours at a time and then conclude by saying: " But this is one of my arcana, which I tell to no one." One of his students would then whisper what he had just said into his ear, and Rovelle would believe that his pupil " had discovered the arcanum by his own sagacity, and would beg him not to divulge what he himself had just told to two hundred persons."

Lombroso has combed history, as it were, with a fine-tooth comb, and very few geniuses have escaped his notice. This paper, so far, is hardly more than a review of his extraordinarily comprehensive work; therefore, I will conclude this portion of it with a list of men of genius, their professions, and their evidences of degeneration, as gathered from his book:

Carlo Dolce, painter, *religious monomania.*

Bacon, philosopher, *megalomania, moral anæsthesia.*

Balzac, writer, *masked epilepsy, megalomania.*

Cæsar, soldier, writer, *epilepsy.*

Beethoven, musician, *amnesia, melancholia.*

Cowper, writer, *melancholia.*

Chateaubriand, writer, *chorea.*

Alexander the Great, soldier, *alcoholism.*

Molière, dramatist, *epilepsy, phthisis pulmonalis.*

Lamb, writer, *alcoholism, melancholia, acute mania.*

Mozart, musician, *epilepsy, hallucinations.*

Heine, writer, *melancholia, spinal disease.*

Dr. Johnson, writer, *chorea.*

Malibran, *epilepsy.*

Newton, philosopher, *amnesia.*

Cavour, statesman, philosopher, *suicidal impulse.*

Ampère, mathematician, *amnesia.*

Thomas Campbell, writer, *chorea.*

Blake, painter, *hallucinations.*

Chopin, musician, *melancholia.*

Coleridge, writer, *alcoholism, morphinism.*

Donizetti, musician, *moral anæsthesia.*

Lenau, writer, *melancholia.*

Mahomet, theologian, *epilepsy.*

Manzoni, statesman, *folie du doute.*

Haller, writer, *hallucinations.*

Dupuytren, surgeon, *suicidal impulse.*

Paganini, musician, *epilepsy.*

Handel, musician, *epilepsy.*

Schiller, writer, *epilepsy.*

Richelieu, statesman, *epilepsy.*

Praga, writer, *alcoholism, sexual perversion.*

Tasso, writer, *alcoholism, melancholia.*

Savonarola, theologian, *hallucinations.*

Luther, theologian, *hallucinations.*

Schopenhauer, philosopher, *melancholia, omniphobia.*

Gogol, writer, *melancholia, tabes dorsalis.*
Lazaretti, theologian, *hallucinations.*
Mallarmé, writer, *suicidal impulse.*
Dostoieffsky, writer, *epilepsy.*
Napoleon, soldier, statesman, *folie du doute, epilepsy.*
Comte, philosopher, *hallucinations.*
Pascal, philosopher, *epilepsy.*
Poushkin, writer, *megalomania.*
Renan, philosopher, *folie du doute.*
Swift, writer, *paresis.*
Socrates, philosopher, *chorea.*
Schumann, musician, *paresis.*
Shelley, writer, *hallucinations.*
Bunyan, writer, *hallucinations.*
Swedenborg, theologian, *hallucinations.*
Loyola, theologian, *hallucinations.*
J. S. Mill, writer, *suicidal impulse.*
Linnæus, botanist, *paresis.*

The reader will observe that I have made use of the comprehensive word, writer, to designate all kinds of literary work except theology and philosophy. The above list is by no means complete, and only contains the names of these geniuses with whom the world is well acquainted.

When we come to the geniuses of the New World, we find that, though few in number, they, nevertheless, show erraticism and degeneration. Poe was undoubtedly a man of great genius, and his degeneration was indicated by his excessive use of alcohol. Aaron Burr was the victim of moral anæsthesia, and Jefferson was pseudo-epileptic and neurasthenic. Randolph was a man of marked eccentricity, and Benedict Arnold was, morally, anæsthetic. Daniel Webster was addicted to an over-indulgence in alcohol, likewise Thomas Marshall and the elder Booth. Booth also had attacks of acute mania. His son Edwin had paresis; so also had John McCullough, John T. Raymond, and Bartley Campbell. A distinguished statesman and politician, and a man who stands high in the councils of the nation, has, for a number of years, given evidence of mental obliquity by his uncontrollable desire for alcohol. No power, outside of bodily restraint, can control him and keep him from indulging his appetite for alcohol when this desire seizes him. One of the most noted poets of to-day, whose verses stir the heart with their pathos and bring smiles to the gravest countenances with their humor, was, for a number of years, an inordinate user of alcohol.

Robert Ingersoll is undoubtedly a man of genius and of considerable originality, and a close study of his writings shows conclusively his mental eccentricity. Judging wholly from his printed utterances, Mr. Ingersoll is only a superficial scientist and mediocre scholar. His power lies in his wonderful word imagery, and his intricately constructed verbal arabesques. He is a verbal symbolist. Symbolism, wherever found, and in whatever art, if carried to any extent, must necessarily be an evidence of atavism, consequently of degeneration.

Thomas Paine gave evidences of a lack of mental equipoise. We find scattered through-

13

out his works the most brilliant, irrefutable,
and logical truths side by side with the most
inane, illogical, and stolid crudities.   Among
other men of genius who showed signs of degeneration we may include Alexander Stevens,
Joel Hart, Adams, Train, Breckenridge, Webster, Blaine, Van Buren, Houston, Grant,
Hawthorne, Bartholow, Walt Whitman.   We
must not confound genius and talent—the two
are widely different.   Genius is essentially
original and spontaneous, while talent is to
some extent acquired.   Genius is a *quasi* abnormality, and one for which the world should
be devoutly grateful.   *Psychos*, in the case of
genius, is not uniformly developed, one part,
being more favored than the others, absorbs
and uses more than its share of that element,
whatsoever it be, which goes to make up intellectuality, hence the less favored or less ac-
quisitive parts show degeneration.

PROPHECY AND INSANITY.

Throughout the whole history of the world a dispassionate survey of prophecy, wherever it is found, shows it always to be engrafted on, or allied with, insanity. In fact this relationship was early recognized, and in many languages the same word is used to designate the prophet and the madman. When the world was young the mind of man was infantile and undeveloped. *Psychos* itself was in its babyhood, and, like a child, exceedingly credulous. Madmen, elevated by maniacal erethism, gave utterance to unheard-of propositions, and men, in their ignorance and credulity, accepted these insane dicta as divine inspirations and made prophets of men who were simply the victims of mental abnormalities. To this day the savage regards the imbecile as the ward of heaven, while all the semi-civilized races of men consider the religious maniac as a holy and authoritative messenger of God!

The Moors declare that the minds of the insane are with God in heaven, and that when they prophesy their every utterance is a direct inspiration. Their holy santons, or prophets, are commonly insane, and are allowed every license. Not long since a newly made bride was ravished by a santon in the city of Tunis, whereupon her husband was congratulated on his good fortune by all his acquaintances. The half insane and wholly bestial priests of the Nairs and kindred races of people in India are invited to the nuptial couch by marriageable maidens, who consider it the greatest honor to yield up their virginity in the embraces of these men of God.

As far back in the past as history reaches we find abundant proof of the toleration and even worship of the religious lunatic. Even in this enlightened age we have our prophets, and even our Christs and Mothers of God, who have their followers and disciples, atavistic congeners of semi-civilized or savage peoples.

The ancient Hebrews used the same word

to designate prophet and madman. We are
told that Saul was weighed down by an evil
spirit and prophesied (raved); in the midst
of this paroxysm he tried to kill David
(homicidal mania). Saul had had attacks before, for we are told that he was seized with
the spirit of prophecy, and astonished his
friends by his vagaries, who asked one another: "Is Saul among the prophets?" Or,
in other words: "Has Saul become insane?"
He had these attacks repeatedly while he was
king, and only the soothing melodies evoked
from the harp of David could calm him.
David feigned madness to escape Achish, who
remarked that he already had as many madmen (*nabi*) about !him as he desired. Here
the word *nabi* (prophet) is used in the sense
of madman.

Some of the prophets of the Old Testament
seem to give evidence of insanity, otherwise
how can we account for their strange vagaries
and nonsensical performances. Hosea married a prostitute because he said God told him

to do so; Ezekiel made a hole in the wall of
his house, through which he removed his fur-
niture instead of through the door; Isaiah
stripped himself naked, and went thus into
the presence of the people; Jeremiah took a
long journey, and at its end hid a linen girdle
in a hole in a rock. He returned home, and
after a time made the same journey and
found the girdle rotten and good for nothing.

This, from a girl of thirteen, resembles some
prophetic visions: "I saw the City of God
from a high tower in its midst. It was beautiful beyond description. The streets were
lined with palaces, and everywhere beautiful
and strange flowers met my eyes. The people
were transported from place to place on
winged carriages. I saw the most beautiful
horses, dogs, cats, and cattle, but all of them
had three heads, two in front and one behind.
As I stood gazing about me I heard a voice
say: 'Take her and set her in the great hall,
and show her the abomination of desolation.'
Immediately I found myself in a great hall

seated on a platform. The hall was filled with people, and these people, both men and women, were naked. They were all playing dominoes. Some of them I knew. I recognized Mr. Cleveland, Mr. Carlisle, Mr. Reed, Mr. Ingalls, Mrs. B., Miss S., Mrs. T., Mr. R., Sallie B., Jennie U., Frank L., and dozens of others. The same voice then said: ' Show her a sign of my wrath.' Straightway a giant angel with ten heads and twenty arms flew through the hall and scattered grains of rice. These grains of rice turned to tigers as I looked, tigers with three heads, which fell upon the people and devoured them. Then the voice said: 'Go tell this to the people, for you are a prophetess and a daughter of God.'"

"You were asleep, Nettie, and dreamed all this."

"No, indeed! I was wide awake. Why, Doctor, I have just this moment come from heaven."

Two thousand years ago this child would

have been considered a prophetess, and divine
honors would have been paid her by her
disciples and followers. Three hundred years
ago she might have had an army at her beck
and call, and, like Joan of Arc, might have
formed a part of the world's history. To-day
science regards her simply as a lunatic; fortunately one that can be cured, for her lunacy
results from mental disorder incident to the
establishment of a natural function peculiar
to her sex, and will disappear sooner or later.

Visions and dreams rule and direct the lives
of all savages, and also in semi-civilized races
these psychical phenomena have great weight.
Joseph was called into the presence of Pharaoh
and treated with great honor because of
his ability to interpret dreams. Everywhere
throughout the whole Bible we find mention
of dreams and visions, and, in fact, some of
the most startling political modifications in
the evolution of the civilized world have been
the direct results of the influence of dreams.
Even at the present time hundreds of en-

lightened and otherwise sane people place the utmost confidence in dreams, and govern their actions accordingly. This is the result of psychical atavism, a reversion back to ancestral beliefs and customs.

Let us now glance at the comparatively recent prophets and saints and see if we can not find marked evidences of insanity in these holy men. It seems strange, yet, nevertheless, it is true, that almost all these saints led (like St. Paul), before their conversions, wild and vicious lives. They thus, by their habits, predisposed their brains to disease. I have only to instance Sts. Anthony, Ignatius Loyola, Juan de Dios, *et al.*, to prove the truth of this assertion.

St. Francis of Assisi was a rake and a spendthrift for twenty-five years of his life. At length his dissolute conduct brought on a severe illness, and he came near dying. When he arose from his sick-bed his entire nature was changed. He wandered about the fields in an aimless manner, sad and sorrowful, sometimes weeping bitterly—a true picture of melancholia. One day he had a vision. He saw Christ nailed to the cross, and he felt, as he declared, "the passion of Christ impressed even on his bowels, upon the very marrow of his bones, so that he could not fix his thoughts upon it without being overflowed with grief." He at length took off his rich clothing and put on the rags of a beggar. Everybody considered him a mad-man, and as such he was driven from pillar to post. With all his madness he was, however, a great and good man. Says Lombroso: "Francis of Assisi, however, was original and great, not through those qualities which he had in common with the vulgar herd of as-cetics—abstinences, mortifications, prayers, ec-stacies, visions—but on account of something which was the very negation of asceticism, without his knowing it—the affirmation and triumph of the gentlest and sweetest feelings of humanity. The ascetic abhorred, con-demned, and fled from nature, life, and all human affections, in order to steep himself in solitary contemplation. Francis, by example and precept, preached the love of nature, concord, mutual affection between human beings, and work. The ascetic called everything beautiful in the world the work of Satan; Francis brought about a true revolution by calling it the work of God, praising and thanking God for it."

San Juan de Dios, early in life, joined the army. The life he led while soldiering had better be imagined than described. He was dismissed from the army for stealing from a comrade. He became a shepherd, and followed this occupation for several years. Finding the quiet life of a shepherd too tame to suit a roystering blade like himself, he reentered the army. After several years' service he became sick, and when he recovered he had lost his memory. He had forgotten even the names of his parents. He again became a shepherd, and soon after began to have hallucinations. He lived for a time in Gibraltar, but, having sold out his little stock of goods, relics, etc., he settled in Granada. Here, while listening to a sermon by Juan d'Avila, he was seized with a sudden maniacal outburst. He confessed his sins with a loud voice, tore his clothing from his body, pulled out his hair by the handful, and rushed through the streets at full speed, imploring God to have mercy on him. He was taken to the Royal Hospital and given the treatment prescribed for lunacy in those days (1539). He was bound with cords and unmercifully flogged in order to drive out the devil or evil spirit supposed to be in possession of him. After his frenzy left him he was released, and he made a vow to go on a pilgrimage to the shrine of the Virgin of Guadalupe.

Notwithstanding the fact that he was without money and that it was in the middle of winter, he started on his pilgrimage, barefoot and clothed in rags. When he arrived at Guadalupe he had a vision " which exercised a decisive influence on him. The

Virgin appeared to him and gave him the Child Jesus, naked, with clothes to cover him. This was to show him that he ought to have pity on the weak, shelter the destitute, and clothe the poor—at least such was his interpretation."

While walking through the city, one day, he saw a sign on a vacant house which read: " House to let for the poor." This gave him the idea of founding an asylum. He begged money from the rich, whom he interested in his scheme, hired and furnished the house, and soon filled it with the sick poor. This was the first free hospital ever inaugurated. The name of this religious lunatic should be revered thoughout all Christendom, for he was the founder of the charity hospital. The doctrine and prophecies of this man are to be admired because of their intense and absolute philanthropy.

Martin Luther had visions and hallucinations. On one occasion, when alone in a certain room which he called his Patmos, he heard nuts moving of their own accord inside a sack and flying round his bed. He thought, too, that showers of berries were thrown at him by invisible hands, whereupon he arose and cried: "Who art thou?" and then commended himself to Christ. On another occasion, when preaching in Wittenberg, he was explaining to his audience the Epistle to the Romans. When he reached the words, "The just shall live by faith," he heard this sentence repeated by a voice several times just at his ear. He had hallucinations of hearing on numerous other occasions, as we learn from his own writings. "Not seldom," writes he, "has it happened to me to awake at midnight and dispute with Satan concerning the mass."

Savonarola had hallucinations of sight and hearing. When he wished to abandon politics and leave them out of his sermons, he heard a voice say, "Fool, dost thou not see that God will have thee go on in the same way?" Says Lombroso, in "The Man of

Genius": "In 1492, while preaching during the Advent, he (Savonarola) had a vision of a sword, on which was written, '*Gladius Domini super terrane*.' Suddenly the sword turned toward the earth, the air was darkened, there was a rain of swords, arrows, and fire, and the earth became a prey to famine and pestilence. From this moment he began to predict the pestilence, which, in fact, afterward came to pass." Savonarola, on another occasion, thought that he went to heaven and held long conversations with the Virgin and many of the saints. He believed that he was the ambassador of Christ and a true prophet!

The insanity of Ste. Jeanne d'Arc is too well known for any comment. I simply introduce her as an example.

Huss was markedly erratic. He had numerous visions, in which he held conversations with angels. Hallucinations of sight and hearing were present in a marked degree.

Mahomet was an epileptic, and his visions and revelations were the result of brain disease. His convulsions are minutely described by contemporaneous Arab writers, and could have been nothing else save epilepsy.

The examples of prophecy and insanity cited in this paper are not introduced in strict chronological order, but appear just as they occurred to the memory of the writer. It can not be denied that these prophets and saints were mentally unbalanced, yet the doctrines they promulgated have been of incalculable benefit to mankind. Most of them preached ethical purity, coincidentally a higher civilization. All were men of genius and of great originality. Genius, no matter in what shape it appears or how erratic it becomes, is sure to lighten the burdens of humanity with some portion of its leaven.

In the process of psychical evolution abstract ethics are the last acquisitions of *psychos*. It frequently happens, however, that disease apparently quickens the perceptions and hurries evolution in some brains, consequently every now and then a prophet springs up who is in advance of his age. He preaches doctrines little understood at the time by the masses. Some few advanced thinkers, and many others who do not think at all, but are only ignorant, consequently credulous, believe in him and follow him. At some future time, long after the death of the prophet, men realize that the ethics he taught, though erratic, were in the main sound and of distinct benefit to the human race. Such were the men whom I have chosen to illustrate this portion of my subject.

On the other hand, there have existed many religious lunatics devoid of *progressive* genius, and who, at best, were but poor imitators of men of genius and originality. Such a one was Joseph Smith, the prophet of the Mormons. This man was the victim of epileptoid seizures. I will quote his own words; he is describing his first vision, which occurred to him after great mental distress and worry. There had been a great religious revival, and he had become very

12

much alarmed. He had gone into the woods
to pray, and while there had been seized
with an *indefinable feeling of terror:* "Just at
this moment of great alarm I saw a pillar of
light, exactly over my head, above the bright-
ness of the sun, which descended gradually
until it fell upon me. It no sooner appeared
than I found myself delivered from the enemy
which held me bound. When the light rested
upon me I saw two personages, whose bright-
ness and glory defy all description, standing
above me in the air. One of them spoke to
me, calling me by name, and said (pointing to
the other), 'This is my beloved son, hear
him.'" After detailing a lengthy conversation which occurred between God and himself, he unconsciously reveals his physical
condition by the following statement: "*When
I came to myself again* I found myself lying on
my back, looking up to heaven." He had
hallucinations of persecution, for, although
only an obscure country lad, fourteen or fifteen
years old, he imagined that men of influence

and standing were persecuting him: "Yet men of high standing would take notice sufficient to excite the public mind against me and create a hot persecution, and this was common among all the sects; all united in persecuting me." Megalomania was also present; he called himself "Joseph, the Seer." The morning after his interview with the Angel Moroni, in which he was shown the place where the Books of Mormon were concealed, he declares that he was utterly exhausted. This is the usual condition of epileptics after a seizure. Smith's scheme of religion, both in the manner in which it was given him by God and its doctrines of polygamy, strikingly resembles that of Mahomet. It is either an imitation or an atavism; in neither case is it conducive to higher civilization.

Swedenborg was probably, to a certain extent, an irresponsible imitator of St. John. The character of his hallucinations tends to show that this was the case in the religious lunacy of this prophet.

Schweinfurth, "the Christ," is a megalo-
maniac and an imitator. His personal appearance indicates degeneration. He is probably
the victim of some form or other of *psychopathia sexualis.*

The founder of the Oneida community of
"perfectionists," John Noyes, was a victim of
psychical atavism and a degenerate. He was
a retrograde prophet, and preached doctrines
which were practiced by our savage ancestors
thousands of years ago. He did not believe
in marriage and the rights of property.
Women, like household goods, he considered
common to the entire community (polyandry
and polygamy); " he did not recognize human
laws, and believed every action, even the
commonest, to be inspired by God."

Throughout all history, both sacred and
profane, wherever we find religious prophecy,
there we are almost certain to find insanity
also.

We discover, also, that there are two kinds
of insane prophets; in the first (progressive

prophets) we find genius and madness combined; in the second (atavistic or retrograde prophets) we find madness with imitation and degeneration.

OCCULTISM, SO-CALLED, THE PHYS-
ICAL RESULT OF MENTAL
INFLUENCES.

The influence of the mind upon the body
has been recognized, in a measure, since the
early history of man; but it is only during the
last decade or so that *psychos* has become an
admitted agent in the production of physical
phenomena heretofore regarded as supernatural and occult. Man has only just begun
to recognize the fact that *psychos* is part and
parcel of his physical organism, and that the
two beings, physical and psychical, are one
and indivisible. Wherever and to whatever
point in the body nerves, nervules, and nerve
filaments penetrate, there *psychos* is to be
found, in some form or other, intimately interwoven and connected with the physical organism.

In the mind are to be found two kinds of
consciousness—a vigilant, coördinating con-

sciousness, and a pseudo-dormant, *unconscious* consciousness. Furthermore, it has been clearly demonstrated that memory is to be found not only in the higher brain centers of the hemispheres, but also in the lower ganglia and even in the nerve filaments governing muscular, venous, and arterial action adjacent to, or remote from, the brain and cord. For convenience, when speaking of consciousness, I will call the first of these two consciousnesses the vigilant consciousness, the second the ganglionic consciousness, and, when speaking of memory, I will differentiate between the two kinds by calling the first conscious memory, and the second ganglionic memory.

Be it observed that I include every mental function in these four psychical operations; I do this both for the sake of brevity and to avoid confusion.

It can be shown, beyond a shadow of doubt, that each and every one of the so-called occult, or supernatural, psychical manifestations to be observed in the *séances* of spiritualists, theosophists, psychicists, averroists, electrobiologists, etc., etc., have their origin in these two consciousnesses and in these two memories.

One of the most familiar, as well as the most frequent, manifestations to be observed at, so-called, spiritual *séances* is table-tipping, table-lifting, table-turning, etc. These phenomena are to be explained by the unconscious influence of expectation on the voluntary muscles. A dozen or so people, fully imbued with the idea that the spirits will move the table, take their places and rest their hands upon it. In a short time, perhaps, agreeable to their expectations, the table begins to move. They have not, voluntarily, exerted a single muscle, but have remained, according to their belief, entirely passive; yet, ganglionic consciousness, influenced by expectation, has exerted stimulation enough on the voluntary muscles of the arms, forearms, and hands to produce a movement of the table.

The movements of Planchette and kindred toys are to be explained in the same way. This involuntary action of the voluntary muscles has been fully demonstrated. An old and well known form of what Peschel would call "shamanism" is the hair, coin and tumbler "spiritualistic" manifestation. A coin is fastened to a hair, which is held in such a manner that the coin is suspended a short distance from the edge or rim of a glass tumbler. The spirits are asked the time of day; the coin, influenced by the unconscious action of the digital muscles, soon begins to oscillate, and will correctly strike the hour on the rim of the tumbler. Bacon was familiar with this experiment, for he says: "There would be a trial made of holding a ring by a thread in a glass, and telling him that holdeth it, before, that it shall strike so many times against the glass and no more."

No one investigated the subject in a scientific manner from the time of Bacon to that of Chevreul. M. Chevreul found that a pendulum affixed by a flexible wire and held by the fingers over mercury would oscillate ; but that when he placed a plate of glass between the mercury and the pendulum the oscillations would cease. He felt sure that the mercury had nothing to do with the oscillations, so fixed the hand holding the wire as well as the arm, and found that the pendulum would not oscillate. He also discovered that with his eyes bandaged a like result followed. He concluded that the oscillations were due to unconscious muscular movement, and that any substance would stop them when placed between the pendulum and the mercury with the *expectation* that they would cease. He remarks that he had a " vague remembrance of being in ' *un etat tout particulier* ' when his eyes followed them (the oscillations)."

Dr. Barrett, of Dublin, has constructed an apparatus so delicate in its adjustments that unconscious muscle movement can easily be shown. An indicator and dial, on which are the letters of the alphabet, connected with a board mounted on wheels, are the essential parts of the machine. The experimenter places his fingers on the board and looks at the lettered dial; he will then think of certain words, and the indicator will at once spell them out on the dial without any conscious volition or movement on his part whatever.

Thought-reading or mind-reading is to be accounted for in the same manner; the involuntary muscle movements of the subject conveying to the so-called mind-reader, who has developed the faculty of reading such movements, a knowledge of the whereabouts of the hidden object. The subject is always told to keep his mind on the object sought for, otherwise the mind-reader invariably fails. In my experiments I have discovered that a tight-fitting glove, a clinching of the hand in the grasp of the performer, or, in fact, any constriction of voluntary action of the muscles in contact with the mind-reader, is sufficient to render his efforts of no avail, even when the sought-for object is kept before the mental vision during the entire time of the experiment.

The varying expressions of the human countenance are produced naturally by no conscious effort. The emotions of joy, sorrow, hate, anger, surprise, etc., express themselves in the muscles of the face through the agency of stimuli affecting ganglionic consciousness. The expectation of experiencing a pleasurable emotion· will depict a corresponding expression on the human countenance without the agency of external stimuli. This is effected through conscious memory and ganglionic consciousness. The unconscious muscle movements of the subject in the hands of the mind-reader are analogous to the involuntary muscle movements produced by the emotions; therefore occultism enters into the one just as much as it enters into the other.

An acquaintance, who is not a professional, and who only practices "mind-reading" for amusement, tells me that his subjects invariably lead him to the neighborhood of the objects sought for by unconscious muscle movements, and that he is enabled to find the objects either by correctly interpreting their movements, or by the involuntary movement of the facial muscles of the bystanders. He also informs me that he has greatly improved by practice, and is now much more expert in "mind-reading" than he was when he first attempted the feat.

It is not my intention to discuss all of the occult forces advanced at various times by different men. They are simply varieties of the same force, therefore I will not enter into any account of odylism, of the odometer of Dr. Mayo, of the magnetometer of Mr. Rutter, and of various other instruments of like character, all of which are but modifications, in point of fact, of Chevreul's pendulum (*pendule explorateure*), and depend on the same occult (!) force, *i. e.*, unconscious and involuntary muscle movement, for their manifestations.

Closely allied to the phenomena just reviewed, and produced by the same cause, *i. e.*,

unconscious muscle movement, is the so-called
occultism, "psychic writing." Last winter I
attended a *séance* conducted by a "first-class
medium," to borrow one of the cant phrases
of those who believe in spiritualism, and, after
the usual table-tipping, table-turning, etc.,
saw "psychic writing" for the first time.

The medium proceeded in the following
manner: She grasped a lead pencil with her
fingers, and held her hand and arm half extended over a pad of writing paper, no portion of her body coming in contact with the
table or writing pad. One of the gentlemen
laid his hand on the back of that of the medium "to complete the psychic circle." In a
few moments the medium's hand began to vibrate and she lowered the pencil to the paper,
where, at first, it made meaningless marks and
scratches, but finally wrote "Dr. W., S——,
S——, S——." I then asked the question:
"Who by the name of S—— wishes to communicate with me?" The reply was: "One
who loves the violin."

A friend of mine, by the name of S——, a violinist of marked ability, died several years ago, and I expressed a belief that it was probably the spirit of this person that wished to communicate with me, whereupon she wrote: "Yes, yes, yes."

This conversation, spoken and written, consumed about ten minutes' time, during which the medium conversed with those about her upon subjects foreign to the matter immediately at hand, nor did she once look at the hand which held the pencil. As far as she was concerned, she had nothing whatever to do with the conscious production of the writings.

I had no reason to believe that the medium had ever seen me before; I am positive that I had never seen nor heard of her until the night in question, and I am equally positive that she did not *voluntarily* write the answers to my questions. Yet, there were the communications, not very long, nor very coherent, it is true, but sufficiently coherent for me to recognize the individual from whom they nominally came. I was convinced that the writing was the result of unconscious muscle movement, but how had her ganglionic consciousness become charged with a knowledge of my musical friend? I puzzled over this question for several days, and finally learned that the medium had lived in my county and had gone to school with an intimate friend of the dead violinist! She had heard her talent discussed hundreds of times, though, in all probability, her active consciousness had entirely forgotten all about the musician at the time of this *séance*.

The medium refused to continue the psychic writing any further during that *séance*, claiming that her arm was tired and painful. I asked the gentleman who had "completed the psychic circle" with the medium, to complete one with me. He did so, and in a few moments, *mirabile dictu, my* hand began to vibrate! This vibration was entirely involuntary on my part and was produced, unques-

tionably, by expectation. I expected that my
hand would vibrate, for I thought that muscle
"fag" produced by the unsupported condition
of the arm would induce vibration. The vibration commenced, however, long before fa-
tigue was felt, so must have been produced
by expectation alone. Before I could experiment any further, refreshments were served (I
believe, designedly), and I lost the opportunity
of showing myself to be a "first-class medium." I have since tried this experiment
repeatedly, and have produced some very
startling results.

An occultism, noticed and commented on
many years ago, has recently been revived in
the person of the "Georgia Wonder," a woman
who goes about the country giving exhibi-
tions of superhuman and marvelous feats of
strength. The woman is described as being
delicate, and non-muscular; yet, showing, at
will, the strength of a dozen strong men.

The fact has long been known that when,
by an effort of the will, the whole energy of

13

the body is concentrated upon some certain
muscular effort, a superhuman, and, I might
say, a supernatural, strength is sometimes
evinced. This is especially noticeable in some
subjects when under the influence of hypnotism. Prof. Carpenter's remarks anent this
portion of the subject are so interesting that I
will quote them : " It was by the artificial in-
duction of a like concentrated effort, coupled
with the assurance of easy success ('it will go
up like a feather'), with which he completely
possessed the subject's mind, that Mr. Braid
(in my presence) enabled a man so remarkable
for the poverty of his physique that he had
not for many years ventured to lift a weight
of twenty pounds, to take up a weight of
twenty-eight pounds upon his little finger, and
swing it around his head with the greatest apparent ease. Neither Mr. Braid nor his son,
both of them powerful men, could do anything
like this; and I could not myself lift the same
weight on my little finger to more than half
my height. Trickery in this case was obvi-

ously impossible; since, if the subject had
been trained to·such feats, the effect of such
training would have been visible in his muscular development."

I have never seen this woman, the " Georgia
Wonder," but from the description of her appearance given me by witnesses who have seen
her, I am inclined to believe that she has the
power of assuming some anomalous form of
hypnotism, and is thus enabled to concentrate
all her energy on some particular muscle effort.
Autohypnotism is by no means infrequent
(*vide* " The Psychology of Hypnotism "),
and its various phases have not yet been
classified, consequently, I regard that form,
through the agency of which this woman per-
forms her feats, as being anomalous. She may
be able, however, by a wonderful exertion of
will power, without the assistance of hypnotism, to call the entire energy of her body to
one or more sets of muscles, and thus evince
superhuman strength. I may support this last

hypothesis by the following instance occurring under my own observation:

A patient of mine had been confined to her bed for many weeks with neurasthenia. One night, while lying in bed, she thought that she heard burglars in the next room, so, getting softly out, she seized a plate chest, containing some seventy or eighty pounds of silver, and carried it down the back stairway, through the yard, out into the alley, and on to the next street, where she dropped it at the feet of a passer-by, and fell completely exhausted. I do not believe that that woman can even lift a like weight now, although she has been restored to health, and now has as much strength as she ever had. Equilibration is likewise an undoubted factor in the "Georgia Wonder's" manifestations.

In reference to that which follows, the reader will bear in mind that I do not restrict the meaning of occultism, but mean it to embrace all those forms of physical and psychical manifestations that are commonly considered pre-ternatural.

A form of occultism is the belief that Christ manifests his presence in the bodies of certain individuals by marks of his wounds, and by causing them to enact the final scenes of his crucifixion and death on the cross. The most celebrated and best known case of stigmatization, as this phenomenon is technically known, is that of Louise Lateau, a young woman of Bois de Haine, Hainaut, Belgium. M. Charbonnier wrote an article on this woman, entitled "*La Maladie des Mystiques: Louise Lateau*," and the Royal Academy of Medicine of Belgium appointed a commission to decide whether or not the paper should appear in one of its publications. The report of this commission (MM. Warlomont and Marcart), embracing observations which extended throughout five months, is very complete, and describes even the most minute details of this remarkable case.

Louise had always been delicate and of

nervous temperament. All her life she had been intensely religious, and it is said of her that long before her first communion: "*Elle savait méditer sur les grands mystères, bien qu' elle n' eût appris de personne la méthode de la méditation. Tout petite, elle aimait à répéter les doux noms de Jésus et de Marie; elle avait une grande dévotion pour la passion du Sauveur, faisait souvent le chemin de la Croix, assistait assidûment à la Sainte Messe, et priait depuis longtemps son chapelet chaque jour.*"

On April 15, 1869, this girl fell into a state of religious ecstacy, during which she saw and conversed with the Virgin Mary and several of the saints. This ecstacy lasted until the 21st of April, when the first of the stigmata made its appearance. Blood oozed from her left side, and, on the following Friday, from her feet also. On the following week blood transuded from the palms of her hands, but not until September 25th did it make its appearance on her forehead. A translated ab-

stract of the commissioners' report reads as
follows:

"Louise passed into a state of ecstacy at an
expected time (Friday), a quarter past 2 o'clock
in the afternoon. Before doing so the pupils
of her eyes were slightly contracted, the eye-
lids almost closed, the eyes expressionless.
When, however, the ecstatic crisis had commenced, the eyes, open and dull, were fixed
upward and directed to the right, the pupils
dilated and almost insensible to light. She
knew nothing of what was going on around
her for a couple of hours. This was the *first*
stage; the *second* was that of genuflection, in
which she clasped her hands and remained in
the attitude of contemplation for a certain
time. A *third* stage was marked by the patient
prostrating herself on the ground without
rigidity. After a while, she made a rapid
movement, the arms were extended in the
form of a cross, and she remained in one attitude for an hour and a half. During the
ecstacy the flow of blood from the stigmata

was considerable; the skin insensible. The entire ecstacy from beginning to end lasted about six hours."

This was undoubtedly a case of autohypnosis, brought on by expectancy, in which the physical phenomena of the stigmata and imitation of the crucifixion were produced by ganglionic consciousness and ganglionic memory. That ganglionic consciousness exerts a powerful effect on the nervous capillaries, no one acquainted with the physiology of the phenomenon of blushing will, for an instant, deny. Vigilant consciousness also, at times, powerfully assists ganglionic consciousness in its influence on the vasomotor nerves. Numerous instances can be cited in which the imagination has produced ecchymoses simulating wounds, and the blood has even transuded from them at times. Dr. Tuke gives the following as a personal observation: "In illustration of the influence of fear or apprehension upon the vascular system, I will give the following example, the case of a highly intelligent lady, well known to myself. Although the emotion had for its object another person, it none the less acted on her own system.

"One day she was walking past a public institution and observed a child in whom she was particularly interested coming out through an iron gate. She saw that he let go the gate after opening it, and it seemed likely to close upon him, and concluded that it would do so with such force as to crush his ankle; however, this did not happen. 'It was impossible,' she says, 'by word or act to be quick enough to meet the supposed emergency; and in fact I found I could not move, for such intense pain came on in the ankle corresponding to the one which I thought the boy would have injured, that I could only put my hand on it to lessen its extreme painfulness. *I am sure I did not move so as to strain or sprain it.* The walk home—the distance of about a quarter of a mile—was very laborious, and in taking off my stocking I found *a circle round the ankle as if it had been painted with red cur-*

rant juice, with a large spot of the same on the outer part. By morning the whole foot was inflamed, and I was a prisoner to my bed for many days.'"

The following instance occurred under my own observation: While attending college, two of my classmates and myself resolved to waylay a lower class man and frighten him. He had walked quite a distance out into the country to see his sweetheart, and we sprang out on him as he was returning to the city. I fired a shot from a revolver straight up into the air. The young man fell at the report of the pistol, crying out that he had been struck in the leg by the bullet and that he was bleeding to death. We carried him to the nearest road-house, and on examination found, on the inner aspect of his right thigh, at the apex of Scarpa's triangle, a round, bright red spot about the size of a silver ten-cent piece, slightly elevated above the skin and very painful. After much persuasion and argument we finally got him to believe that he had not been shot, though none of us could explain the presence of the spot. The stigma disappeared in a day or so without giving him further trouble.

Before dismissing the subject of stigmatization, I may say that two cases have come under my personal observation. One of the cases, that of Mrs. Stutzenburg, of Louisville, Ky., I examined only casually, those in charge of her not allowing me to approach her or to examine the stigmata. I have it on good authority, however, that the woman was a fraud and produced the bloody spots artificially. The other instance, strange to say, occurred in a Jewess, and was a genuine case of stigmatization. The young girl was exceedingly hysterical and had been under my care for some time. She had an intimate friend, a devout Catholic, who had succeeded in converting her to Christianity. I only saw her twice after the appearance of the stigmata, which presented the appearance of ecchymoses, the one over the heart being triangular in shape; those on the backs of her hands and feet being spherical and ovoid; those in the palms of the hands and on the bottoms of the feet being linear. She was removed from the city shortly after the appearance of the stigmata, and died, I understand, soon after her removal.

In the majority of instances of clairvoyance, second-sight, etc., given by believers in this form of occultism, the facts in the case are greatly distorted, or, very frequently, are manufactured to suit the occasion. When not to be accounted for by suggestion and expectancy, they fall under the law of coincidences. There *is* a law of coincidences, theoretical, it is true, yet no more so than the law of deviation from an average; and M. Chetelet's tables will apply as well to one as to the other.

One night, after a hard and very fatiguing day's work at the microscope, I had some difficulty in going to sleep. At length I lost consciousness, when suddenly I heard the sentence, "He is dead!" whispered in my ear.

I seemed to ask the question, "Who is dead?" and was awakened by the answer, seemingly shouted in loud tones: "Paul Volofsky." I passed an hour trying to recall where I had heard, if ever, this name, but was unable to do so. The next morning, while reading a newspaper, I saw that Paul Volofsky had been killed in a street fight at 1 o'clock on the previous night. I tried again to remember when I had heard, if ever, the name of Paul Volofsky, but all in vain. I then went to the morgue (this occurred in New York), and took a look at the dead man.

As soon as I saw the face, I remembered at once when I had seen him and where I had heard his name. Several days before the occurrence of these events I had occasion to cash a check at a down-town bank, and the man who was at the teller's window before my turn came was this man, and I heard him give his name in reply to a question put to him by the teller. When he turned to go, I glanced at his face, and remembered it at once

when I saw it again in the morgue. The day
on which I was at the bank, I was in a great
hurry, and the man's slowness and obtuseness
in understanding the explanations of the
teller aggravated my impatience, consequently
his name impressed itself superficially on my
memory, and deeply on my ganglionic memory. At a time when vigilant consciousness
and conscious memory were lost in sleep, ganglionic memory resurrected this name. The
fact that the man was killed that night I regard simply as a coincidence.

Again, a friend of mine, who has a very
peculiar name, once went to see a celebrated
clairvoyant. He mentioned his name during
the conversation that ensued, and the woman
remarked on its peculiarity, saying that she
had never heard a name like his before. She
hypnotized herself, and immediately commenced a thrilling tale of a steamboat fire in
which my friend lost his life. It so happens
that, five years before this *séance*, a man having
exactly the same name as that of my friend

was burned to death during the conflagration of a New Orleans packet, and that the horror of his terrible death was fully detailed in the newspapers of that date. The ganglionic consciousness of the woman had retained the details of this disaster throughout the five intervening years; the strange name, heard again after many years, had aroused ganglionic memory; autohypnosis had locked up vigilant consciousness and conscious memory, so out came the story just as the woman had read it five years before!

Although I will not call that false which I have not investigated and found to be untrue, I feel perfectly safe in saying that all tales of clairvoyance, of levitation, of Thibetan occultism should be taken *cum grano salis*. When subjected to true scientific investigation, I firmly and unquestionably believe that they will prove to be produced by no truer occult force than that which swayed *la pendule explorateure* in the hands of M. Chevreul!

THE EFFECT OF FEMALE SUFFRAGE ON POSTERITY.

The greatest, best, and highest law of higher civilization is that which declares that man should strive to benefit, not himself alone, but his posterity.

I. THE ORIGIN OF THE MATRIARCHATE.

In the very beginning woman was, by function, a mother; by virtue of her surroundings, a housewife. Man was then, as now, the active, dominant factor in those affairs outside the immediate pale of the fireside. Life was collective; "communal was the habitation, and communal the wives with the children; the men pursued the same prey, and devoured it together after the manner of wolves; all felt, all thought, all acted in concert." Primitive men were like their simian ancestors, which never paired, and which roamed through the forests in bands and troops. This collectivism is plainly noticeable in certain races of primitive folks which are yet in existence, notably the autochthons of the Aleutian Islands. Huddled together in their communal *kachims*, naked, without any thought of immodesty, men, women, and children share the same fire and eat from the same pot. They recognize no immorality in the fact of the father cohabiting with his daughter—one of them naïvely remarking to Langsdorf, who reproached him for having committed this crime: "Why not? the otters do it!" Later in life the men and women mate; but even then there is no sanctity in the marriage tie, for the Aleutian will freely offer his wife to the stranger within his gates, and will consider it an insult if he refuses to enjoy her company. "As with many savages and half-civilized people, the man who would not offer his guest the hospitality of the conjugal couch, or the company of his best-looking daughter, would be considered an ill-bred person."

This laxity in sexual relations was, at first,

16

common to all races of primitive men, but, after a time, there arose certain influences which modified, to a certain extent, this free and indiscriminate intercourse. Frequent wars must have occurred between hostile tribes of primitive men, during which, some of them (physically or numerically weaker than their opponents) must have been repeatedly vanquished, and many of their females captured, for, in those old days (like those of more recent times, for that matter) the women were the prizes for which the men fought.

Under circumstances like these, the few remaining women must have served as wives for all the men of the tribe; and, in this manner polyandry had its inception. Polyandry gives women certain privileges which monandry denies, and she is not slow to seize on these prerogatives, and to use them in the furtherance of her own welfare. Polyandry, originating from any cause whatever, will always end in the establishment of a matriarchate, in which the women are either directly or indirectly at the head of the government.

There are several matriarchates still extant in the world, and one of the best known, as well as the most advanced, as far as civilization and culture are concerned, is that of the Nairs, a people of India inhabiting that portion of the country lying between Cape Comorin and Mangalore, and the Ghâts and the Indian Ocean.

The Nairs are described as being the handsomest people in the world; the men being tall, sinewy and extraordinarily agile, while the women are slender and graceful, with perfectly modeled figures. The Nair girl is carefully chaperoned until she arrives at a marriageable age, say, fourteen or fifteen years, at which time some complaisant individual is selected, who goes through the marriage ceremony with her. As soon as the groom ties the *tali*, or marriage cord, about her neck, he is feasted and is then dismissed; the wife must never again speak to, or even look at, her husband. Once safely wedded, the girl becomes emancipated, and can receive the attentions of as many men as she may elect, though, I am informed, it is not considered fashionable, at present, to have more than seven husbands, one for each day of the week.

Of no importance heretofore, after her farcical marriage the Nair woman at once becomes a power in the councils of the nation; as a matter of course, the higher her lovers the higher her rank becomes and the greater her influence. Here is female suffrage in its primitive form, brought about, it is true, by environment, and not by elective franchise.

As far as the children are concerned, the power of the mother is absolute; for they know no father, the maternal uncle standing in his stead. Property, both personal and real, is vested in the woman; she is the mistress and the ruler. "The mother reigns and governs; she has her eldest daughter for prime minister in her household, through whom all orders are transmitted to her little world.

Formerly, in grand ceremonials, the reigning prince himself yielded precedence to his eldest daughter, and, of course, recognized still more humbly the priority of his mother, before whom he did not venture to seat himself until she had given him permission. Such was the rule from the palace to the humblest dwelling of a Nair."

During the past fifty years, these people have made rapid strides toward civilization, monandry and monogamy taking the places of polyandry and polygamy, and fifty or a hundred years hence, this matriarchate will, in all probability, entirely disappear.

I have demonstrated, I think, clearly and distinctly, that matriarchy, or female government, is neither new nor advanced thought, but that it is as old, almost, as the human race; that the "New Woman" was born many thousands of years ago, and that her autotype, in some respects, is to be found to-day in Mangalore! A return to matriarchy at the present time would be distinctly and

emphatically and essentially retrograde in
every particular. The right to vote carries
with it the right to hold office, and if women
are granted the privilege of suffrage, they
must also be given the right to govern. Now
let us see if we can not find a reason for this
atavistic desire (matriarchy) in the physical
and psychical histories of its foremost advocates. I will discuss this question in Part II
of this paper.

II. The Viragint.

There are two kinds of genius. The first is
progressive genius, which always enunciates
new and original matter of material benefit to
the human race, and which is, consequently,
non-atavistic; the second is atavistic or retrogressive genius, which is imitative, and which
always enunciates dead and obsolete matter
long since abandoned and thrown aside as
being utterly useless. The doctrines of communism and of nihilism are the products of
retrogressive genius and are clearly atavistic,

inasmuch as they are a reversion to the
mental habitudes of our savage ancestors.
The doctrines of the matriarchate are likewise
degenerate beliefs, and, if held by any civilized being of to-day, are evidences of psychic
atavism.

Atavism invariably attacks the weak; and
individuals of neurasthenic type are more frequently its victims than are any other class of
people. Especially is this true in the case of
those who suffer from psychical atavism.

The woman of to-day who believes in and
inculcates the doctrines of matriarchy, doctrines which have been, as far as the civilized
world is concerned, thrown aside and abandoned these many hundred years, is as much
the victim of psychic atavism as was Alice
Mitchell, who slew Freda Ward in Memphis
several years ago, and who was justly declared a viragint by the court that tried her.

Without entering into the truthfulness or
falseness of the theory advanced by me
elsewhere in this book, in regard to the

primal cause of psychic hermaphroditism, which I attributed and do still attribute to psychic atavism, I think that I am perfectly safe in asserting that every woman who has been at all prominent in advancing the cause of equal rights in its entirety, has either given evidences of masculo-femininity (viraginity), or has shown, conclusively, that she was the victim of psycho-sexual aberrancy. Moreover, the history of every viragint of any note in the history of the world shows that they were either physically or psychically degenerate, or both.

Jeanne d'Arc was the victim of hystero-epilepsy, while Catharine the Great was a dipsomaniac, and a creature of unbounded and inordinate sensuality. Messalina, the depraved wife of Claudius, a woman of masculine type, whose very form embodied and shadowed forth the regnant idea of her mind—absolute and utter rulership—was a woman of such gross carnality, that her lecherous conduct shocked even the depraved courtiers of her lewd and salacious court. The side-lights of history, as Douglas Campbell has so cleverly pointed out in his "Puritan in Holland, England, and America," declare that there is every reason to believe that the Virgin Queen, Elizabeth of England, was not such a pure and unspotted virgin as her admirers make her out to be. Sir Robert Cecil says of her that "she was more man than woman," while history shows conclusively that she was a pronounced viragint, with a slight tendency toward megalomania. In a recent letter to me, Mr. George H. Yeaman, ex-Minister to Denmark, writes as follows : " Whether it be the relation of cause and effect, or only what logicians call a " mere coincidence," the fact remains that in Rome, Russia, France, and England, political corruption, cruelty of government, sexual immorality—nay, downright, impudent, open, boastful indecency—have culminated, for the most part, in the eras of the influence of viragints on government or over governors."

Viraginity has many phases. We see a mild form of it in the tom-boy who abandons her dolls and female companions for the marbles and masculine sports of her boy acquaintances. In the loud-talking, long-stepping, slang-using young woman we see another form; while the square-shouldered, stolid, cold, unemotional, unfeminine android (for she has the normal human form, without the normal human *psychos*) is yet another. The most aggravated form of viraginity is that known as homo-sexuality; with this form, however, this paper has nothing to do.

Another form of viraginity is technically known as gynandry, and may be defined as follows: A victim of gynandry not only has the feelings and desires of a man, but also the skeletal form, features, voice, etc., so that the individual approaches the opposite sex anthropologically, and in more than a psycho-sexual way (Krafft-Ebing).

As it is probable that this form of viraginity is sometimes acquired to a certain ex-

tent, and that, too, very quickly, when a
woman is placed among the proper surroundings, I shall give the case of Sarolta, Countess
V., one of the most remarkable instances
of gynandry on record. If this woman, when
a child, had been treated as a girl, she would
in all probability have gone through life as
a woman, for she was born a female in every
sense of the word. At a very early age,
however, her father, who was an exceedingly
eccentric nobleman, dressed her in boy's clothing, called her Sandor, and taught her boyish
games and sports.

"Sarolta-Sandor remained under her father's influence till her twelfth year, and then
came under the care of her maternal grand-
mother, in Dresden, by whom, when the masculine play became too obvious, she was placed
in an institute and made to wear female attire.
At thirteen she had a love relation with an
English girl, to whom she represented herself
as a boy, and ran away with her. She was
finally returned to her mother, who could do

nothing with her, and was forced to allow her
to resume the name of Sandor and to put on
boy's clothes.   She accompanied her father on
long journeys, always as a young gentleman;
she became a *roué*, frequenting brothels and
cafés and often becoming intoxicated.   All of
her sports were masculine; so were her tastes
and so were her desires.   She had many love
affairs with women, always skillfully hiding
the fact that she herself was a woman.   She
even carried her masquerade so far as to enter
into matrimony with the daughter of a distinguished official and to live with her for
some time before the imposition was discovered."   The woman whom Sandor married is
described as being " a girl of incredible sim-
plicity and innocence;" in sooth, she must
have been!

Notwithstanding this woman's passion for
those of her own sex, she distinctly states
that in her thirteenth year she experienced
normal sexual desire.   Her environments,
however, had been those of a male instead

of a female, consequently her psychical weakness, occasioned by degeneration inherited from an eccentric father, turned her into the gulf of viraginity, from which she at last emerged, a victim of complete gynandry. I have given this instance more prominence than it really deserves, simply because I wish to call attention to the fact that environment is one of the great factors in evolutionary development.

Many women of to-day who are in favor of female suffrage are influenced by a single idea; they have some great reform in view, such as the establishment of universal temperance, or the elevation of social morals. Suffrage in its entirety, that suffrage which will give them a share in the government, is not desired by them; they do not belong to the class of viragints, unsexed individuals, whose main object is the establishment of a matriarchate.

Woman is a creature of the emotions, of impulses, of sentiment, and of feeling; in her the logical faculty is subordinate. She is influenced by the object immediately in view, and does not hesitate to form a judgment which is based on no other grounds save those of intuition. Logical men look beyond the immediate effects of an action and predicate its results on posterity. The percepts and recepts which form the concept of equal rights also embody an eject which, though conjectural, is yet capable of logical demonstration, and which declares that the final and ultimate effect of female suffrage on posterity would be exceedingly harmful.

We have seen that the pronounced advocates and chief promoters of equal rights are probably viragints—individuals who plainly show that they are psychically abnormal; furthermore, we have seen that the abnormality is occasioned by degeneration, either acquired or inherent, in the individual. Now let us see, if the right of female suffrage were allowed, what effect it would produce on the present environment of the woman of to-day, and, if any, what effect this changed

environment would have on the psychical
habitudes of the woman of the future. This
portion of the subject will be discussed in
Part III of this paper.

III. The Decadence.

It is conceded that man completed his cycle
of physical development many thousands of
years ago. Since his evolution from his pithecoid ancestor the forces of nature have been
at work evolving man's psychical being. Now,
man's psychical being is intimately connected
with, and dependent upon, his physical being ;
therefore it follows that degeneration of his
physical organism will necessarily engender
psychical degeneration also. Hence, if I can
prove that woman, by leading a life in which
her present environments are changed, produces physical degeneration, it will naturally
follow that psychical degeneration will also
accrue ; and, since one of the invariable results
of degeneration, both physical and psychical,
is atavism, the phenomenon of a social revolu-

tion in which the present form of government will be overthrown and matriarchy established in its stead, will be not a possibility of the future, but a probability.

That the leaders of this movement in favor of equal rights look for such a result, I have not the slightest doubt; for, not many days ago, Susan B. Anthony stood beside the chair of a circuit judge in one of our court-houses and, before taking her seat, remarked that there were those in her audience who doubtless thought "that she was guilty of presumption and usurpation," but that there would come a day when they would no longer think so!

Statistics show clearly and conclusively that there is an alarming increase of suicide and insanity among women, and I attribute this wholly to the already changed environment of our women. As the matter stands they have already too much liberty. The restraining influences which formerly made woman peculiarly a housewife have been, in

a measure, removed, and woman mixes freely
with the world. Any new duty added to
woman as a member of society would modify
her environment to some extent and call for
increased nervous activity. When a duty
like suffrage is added the change in her environment must necessarily be marked and
radical, with great demands for increased activity. The right of suffrage would, unquestionably, very materially change the environment of woman at the present time, and
would entail new and additional desires and
emotions which would be other and most
exhausting draughts on her nervous organism.

The effects of degeneration are slow in
making their appearance, yet they are exceedingly certain. The longer woman lived amid
surroundings calling for increased nervous
expenditure, the greater would be the effects
of the accruing degeneration on her posterity.
"Periods of moral decadence in the life of a
people are always contemporaneous with

17

times of effeminacy, sensuality, and luxury. These conditions can only be conceived as occurring with increased demands on the nervous system, which must meet these requirements. As a result of increase of nervousness there is increase of sensuality, and since this leads to excess among the masses it undermines the foundations of society — the morality and purity of family life" (Krafft-Ebing).

The inherited psychical habitudes, handed down through hundreds and thousands of years, would prevent the immediate destruction of that ethical purity for which woman is noted, and in the possession of which she stands so far above man. I do not think that this ethical purity would be lost in a day or a year, or a hundred years, for that matter; yet there would come a time when the morality of to-day would be utterly lost, and society would sink into some such state of existence as we now find *en evidence* among the Nairs. In support of this proposition I have only to instance the doctrines promulgated by some of the most advanced advocates of equal rights. The "free love" of some advanced women, I take it, is but the free choice doctrine in vogue among the Nairs and kindred races of people.

John Noyes, of the Oneida Community, where equal rights were observed, preached the same doctrines. It is true that the people who advocate such unethical principles are degenerate individuals, psychical atavists, yet they faithfully foreshadow in their own persons that which would be common to all men and women at some time in the future, if equal rights were allowed, and carried out in their entirety.

This is an era of luxury, and it is a universally acknowledged fact that luxury is one of the prime factors in the production of degeneration. We see forms and phases of degeneration thickly scattered throughout all circles of society, in the plays which we see performed in our theaters, and in the books and papers published daily throughout the land. The greater portion of the *clientèle* of the alienist and neurologist is made up of women who are suffering with neurotic troubles, generally of a psychopathic nature. The number of viragints, gynandrists, androgynes, and other psycho-sexual aberrants of the feminine gender is very large indeed.

It is folly to deny the fact that the right of female suffrage will make no change in the environment of woman. The New Woman glories in the fact, that the era which she hopes to inaugurate will introduce her into a new world. Not satisfied with the liberty she now enjoys, and which is proving to be exceedingly harmful to her in more ways than one, she longs for more freedom, a broader field of action. If nature provided men and women with an inexhaustible supply of nervous energy, they might set aside physical laws, and burn the candle at both ends without any fear of its being burned up. Nature furnishes each individual with just so much nervous force and no more; moreover, she holds every one strictly accountable for every portion of nervous energy which he or she may squander; therefore, it behooves us to build our causeway with exceeding care, otherwise we will leave a chasm which will engulf posterity.

The baneful effects resulting from female suffrage will not be seen to-morrow, or next week, or week after next, or next month, or next year, or a hundred years hence, perhaps. It is not a question of our day and generation; it is a matter involving posterity. The simple right to vote carries with it no immediate danger, the danger comes afterward; probably many years after the establishment of female suffrage, when woman, owing to her increased degeneration, gives free rein to her atavistic tendencies, and hurries ever backward toward the savage state of her barbarian ancestors. I see, in the establishment of equal rights, the first step toward that abyss of im-

moral horrors so repugnant to our cultivated
ethical tastes—the matriarchate. Sunk as
low as this, civilized man will sink still lower
—to the communal *kachims* of the Aleutian
Islanders.

ANIMISM AND THE RESURRECTION.

The belief in the existence of the soul, and consequent resurrection or re-animation of the body after death, was evolved in the mind of man very early in his history. It is, comparatively speaking, very easy to trace out in the burial ceremonies and beliefs as shown in the relics of primitive races that still exist, and of those races now extinct, but which have left lasting evidences of their funeral rites on their monuments and in their graves, the origin of animism or the belief in ghosts or souls. I do not wish to appear prolix, but, in order to present clearly and succinctly the theory of the origin of the belief in the resurrection of the body, it will be necessary to give a detailed account of the burial ceremonies and the peculiar beliefs of certain peoples who were, and are, primitive folk. I then wish to show that the present belief in the resurrection of the body is simply an atavism; a reversion back to the primitive beliefs of our savage ancestors. Before entering on this, however, it will be proper to trace out the origin of religion, and to show, incidentally, that a belief or a non-belief in the existence of the soul is, primarily, the fundamental basis of the acquired ethical emotion —religion.

When man had reached a mental acuteness that enabled him to use weapons and traps in securing his food, his struggle for existence became easy, and he began to notice and to inquire into the various natural phenomena by which he was surrounded. He soon discovered that his prosperity was governed by Nature, and ended by creating a system of theogony founded entirely on natural objects and natural phenomena. He gave to the sun, the moon, the stars, the thunder, the wind; to mountains, hills, and dales, to volcanoes, water-falls, and floods, distinct personalities. He regarded them as beings like himself, only much more powerful; beings that he must propitiate in order to gain their good-will. His worship and devotion, however, was like that of the dog which creeps to your feet on its belly when it wishes to gain your good-will. It had no ethical element in it whatever and very little, if any, of the spiritual. The idea of the spiritual was evolved later on.

It will be observed that I make Nature-worship the first religion of man. This is contrary to the views of Spencer, Taylor, and others, who regard animism, or ancestral worship, as man's first religion.

In those races in which ancestral worship is to be found, we find vestiges of the still older religion — Nature-worship, interwoven and commingling with it, and, as a matter of course, with the last religion acquired showing the most prominence.

We see in the genesis of man, as given by almost every one of the primitive races, that man himself sprang from the sun or the moon or some other natural object. I have only to refer to the genesis of the human race (their own

of course) as declared by the Aztecs (Biart),
the Peruvians (Prescott), the Aleutians (Reclus), the Ainus of Japan (Batchelor), the
Ishogos (Müller), the North American Indians
(Bancroft), the Inoits (Reclus), the Indians of
Yucatan (Stevens), and numerous other primitive folk, to show that Nature, or some object
in Nature, was regarded as the creator. Even
the omnipotent Unkulunkulu of the Amazulu,
"who sprang up from a bed of reeds," and
whom Spencer uses to clinch his theory of
the priority of animism in religion, bears a
striking resemblance to that "fair white warrior" (the sun god) of the Caribs, who "sprang
up from his bed in the eastern sea."

Says Spencer in his "Principles of Sociology: "Leaving unsettled the question
whether there are men in whom dreams have
not generated the notion of a double, and the
sequent notion that at death the double has
gone away, we may hold it as settled that the
first conception of a supernatural being is the
conception of a ghost." This I do not believe.

Facts, gathered from the legends, myths, and folk-lore of primitive peoples, as well as actual observation, do not warrant any such conclusion.

The ancient Hebrews, the chosen people of God, according to their belief, had no belief in the existence of ghosts or souls, yet they had their gods (*elohim*), and their angels, beings eminently supernatural. I fail to find in the writings of Moses, or, rather, in the writings attributed to Moses, any reference to the immortality of the human soul; nor do I find any vestiges of ancestral worship, yet these people had an overweening respect for their progenitors. Their prayers were always directed to the God of Abraham, Isaac, and Jacob, and not to the patriarchs themselves. I do find, however, numerous relics and reminders of Nature-worship, and Phallic worship, the direct offspring of solar worship.

During their captivity, the Israelites acquired some idea of Satan and hell (*Sheitan* and *sheol*) from their conquerors, yet some of them believed in the non-existence of the soul up to, and after, the crucifixion of Christ.

Numerous tribes of Indians in North and South America, when first discovered, as we gather from the testimony of Balboa, Garcilasso, Junipero Serra, Ovendano, and many others, had no idea of ghost or soul and did not worship anything, yet they looked upon the phenomena of Nature with awe, and, some of them at least, had even evolved, to a slight extent, the idea of propitiation.

Mr. Bond, an English engineer, some time since asserted that he had found the missing ape-man in the mountains of the Western Ghauts. In speaking of their religious belief, he says: "These people have no words in their vocabulary for ghost, spirit, devil, or god. They seem to worship Nature." When Magellan discovered the Tierra del Fuegians, he found them without any religious beliefs whatever, yet with a shadowy awe of the phenomena of Nature. "The

Dacotahs never pray to the creator; if they wish for fine weather, they pray to the weather itself," says Lubbock. I might give dozens of other instances in support of the priority of Nature-worship, but deem it hardly necessary.

Man lived in the world thousands of years worshiping or propitiating Nature before he arrived at that degree of psychical development necessary to evolve an idea of ghost or soul. When his struggle for existence, owing to his increased mental sagacity, became easy, he had time to study the psychical phenomena belonging to his own personal being. He began to notice that while he slept he would go out on a hunting expedition, and experience numerous adventures; or that he would visit strange places; or that he would see and converse with his dead relatives and friends.

He at length evolved the idea that he had a double, and that this double left him on occasions. Again, he noticed that after a swoon, in which his comrade appeared to sleep, his double came back to him again; or, after profound coma, the result of wounds or blows, this same thing sometimes occurred. Says Spencer: "He witnesses insensibilities various in their degrees. After the immense majority of them there come reanimations—daily after sleep, frequently after a swoon, occasionally after coma, now and then after wounds and blows. What about this other form of insensibility?—will not reanimation follow this also? The inference that it will is strengthened by the occasional experience that revival occurs unexpectedly. One, in course of being buried, suddenly comes back to himself. The savage does not take this for proof that the man supposed to be dead was not dead; but it helps to convince him that the insensibility of death is like all the other insensibilities."

What wonder, then, that this confusion should exist; and that it does exist there can be no doubt. The Bushmen say, "Death is only a sleep." In 1889 an Ishogo, newly arrived from Africa, sang me a funeral song, which may be translated as follows: "Sleep on, beloved, the cattle are in the kraal and the plantains are plucked for to-morrow's feast. Wake thou in the morning when the funeral drums beat, or, if thou wakest not, go thou to Mbataka, the place [home] of the dead." The Tasmanians stick a spear in the grave of the dead man " to fight with while he sleeps," as one of them told Bonwick. "When a Toda dies the people entertain a lingering hope that, till putrefaction commences, reanimation may possibly take place." The dead body of a Damara is sewn up in a bullock's hide and buried; the people then jump to and fro over the grave to keep the dead man from rising out of it. The Tupis tie the limbs of the dead man with cords, so that he may not get out and trouble his friends with untimely visits. Some races endeavor to bring back the departing or departed soul and cause it to reanimate the body. The Chinese ring bells and beat gongs in the yards and streets adjacent to the houses of the sick, in order to frighten back the departing souls into their earthly tenements. According to Alexander, the Arawaks flagellate the bodies of the dead in the hope of reanimating them; the Hottentots indulge in a similar practice.

In 1636, that portion of Canada lying between Georgian Bay, Lake Huron, and Lake Simcoe, and which is bounded on the north by the River Severn, was occupied by a powerful tribe of Indians called Hurons. In recent times several enormous accumulations of human bones have been discovered in this section of the country. These heaps of bones have puzzled more than one scientist, who has been at a loss to account for them. "Among those who have wondered and speculated over these remains," says Francis Parkman, "is Mr. Schoolcraft. A slight acquaintance with the early writers would have solved his doubts." Bribeuf, a Jesuit priest, who was stationed in Canada and who visited these Indians in 1636, has left us a clear record, in his "Relations des Hurons," of the origin of these ossuaries. He gives us, in this plain matter-of-fact story, a minute and exact description of the burial rites of these primitive people. Charlevoix, Bressani, Du Creux, and Lafitau have likewise left us interesting histories of the mortuary ceremonies of these autochthons.

When a Huron departed this life his corpse was placed, in a sitting posture, in the center of his wigwam. His relations and friends then took places around him and bewailed his taking off, imploring him to return and not to leave them. Laudatory speeches were made to him by the chiefs and others in authority. The corpse was invariably treated with great respect, for these people believed that it was still the dwelling-place of the soul. After a day or two spent in ceremonies like these, the relations wrapped the body in furs, first placing his spear, his bow, and his toma-

18

hawk by his side, and then deposited the
body on a scaffold in the outskirts of the village. Every twelve years the bodies that had
accumulated were taken down from the scaf-
folds and prepared for their final interment
in the common ossuary of the tribe. The
furs were unwrapped and the bones of the
dead individuals exposed. These bones were
tenderly caressed and fondled by the women,
who uttered loud cries of woe and lamenta-
tion. Says Bribeuf: "*J'admiray la tendresse
d'une femme son pere et ses enfans; elle est fille
d'un capitaine (chief), qui est mort fort agé,
et a esté autre fois fort considerable dans le
pais; elle luy peignoit sa chevaleure, elle manoit
ses os les uns après les autres, avec la mesme
affection qui ai elle luy eust voulu rendre la
vie oct.*" They considered that these bones
were sentient and still occupied by the soul.
These grisly remains were finally tied in
bundles and carried to the place of final
sepulture, the inhabitants of each town starting at the same time, all converging toward

this central ossuary. When all had arrived
with their gruesome burdens a feast was held,
gifts were distributed and the bones deposited in an immense pit, along with large
copper kettles filled with food, and the whole
covered with earth. Not until this last ceremony, so the Indians thought, did the soul
abandon the body and journey to the spirit
world. Almost all of the aboriginal tribes
of North America had beliefs analogous to
those held by the Hurons. They may have
differed in non-essential points, but, taken all
in all, their beliefs were identical.

As the mind of man developed, he acquired
a new insight into the phenomena of death,
consequently his funeral rites, ceremonies, and
beliefs underwent modification. He lost the
idea of reanimation and acquired that of
future resurrection. This is not true of all
men, for some races of men gave up the idea
of resurrection in its entirety; for instance,
the Semitic and Indo-European races. Other
races also abandoned this idea, but it is not

necessary to enumerate them here. The
Egyptians, however, held to this modified
view of the resurrection, as is clearly indicated
by the care they manifested in mummifying
the remains of their dead. Inscriptions on
their monuments and on the mummy-cases
themselves also disclose this.

Primarily, food, raiment, weapons, etc.,
were placed by the corpse in the hope of an
immediate reanimation. They were placed
there to be used by the man himself when his
double came back, and he awoke from his insensibility. Time, however, changed the significance of these offerings; they at length
became offerings, not to the man himself, but
to his ghost or spirit. Not only did the savage arrive at the idea of a human soul, but
he became imbued with the idea that not
only all animals had souls, but that even in-
animate objects had them likewise. This is
clearly indicated by the contents of neo-
sepultural mounds, dolmens, cromlechs, and
tombs, and also by the funeral ceremonies of

some of the modern savages. In these, comparatively speaking, recent tombs the bowls, vases, cups, and weapons are found broken in pieces—so broken that their souls might accompany their dead owner to the spirit-world. In the most ancient graves the utensils are always intact, thus showing that the universal-soul idea had not been evolved. At the time of Christ, the whole civilized world had abandoned the idea of a bodily resurrection. It had been relegated to that depository of so many savage crudities—absolute oblivion. Now let us glance for one instant at its revival.

In another paper (see " Genius and Degeneration") I think that I have clearly demonstrated that genius is always accompanied by degeneration, and that this degeneration may be either physical or psychical, or both combined. Now degeneration and atavism are synonymous terms; wherever there is atavism or reversion there is likewise degeneration. St. Paul, the great exponent of the resurrection of the body, was a man of transcendant genius. He taught the grandest, most sublime, and divinest philosophy ever enunciated by the lips of man. Nature never errs in her fundamental laws, therefore one would expect to find, necessarily, some evidences of degeneration in a great genius like Paul, and we are not disappointed in this expectation.

He himself speaks of "his thorn in the flesh," which, from the character of his seizure while traveling on the Damascus road, I think, beyond the shadow of a doubt, was true epilepsy. We would naturally expect to find psychical degeneration also in a man afflicted with a disease like epilepsy, and we do find it in his belief in the resurrection of the body, a belief formulated by the immature minds of men in the very beginning of their psychical existence, and thrown aside by them as absurd as soon as their enlightened intelligence taught them otherwise. The Hebrews had abandoned this belief long before the time of Moses, and had even abandoned all belief in the immortality of the soul. They had reacquired the latter belief during their captivity, and at the time of Christ believed (that is, a majority of them did,) in Sheol, a place analogous to the Hades of the Latins. The Sadducees did not believe in the immortality of the soul, but thought that it became extinct along with life at death. The belief in the resurrection of the body, since the time of Christ, has been mainly a matter of education, people accepting it as a doctrinal *sine qua non* without giving it one thought, one way or the other. At the present time, however, quite a number of Christians reject it, and consider the idea as wholly untenable. When we pause and consider that the greatest exponent of this doctrine was probably an epileptic, and that the doctrine itself is patently an instance of psychical atavism, ought we to wonder that they do?

SUICIDE IN THE UNITED STATES.

This paper has been prepared with special reference to suicide as observed in the United States, though voluntary death as found throughout the entire world is, incidentally, discussed therein.

Self-slaughter is of rare occurrence among savage races of people; of so infrequent occurrence, in fact, that one is almost tempted to say that it is unknown among them. This would be, however, a statement not authorized by facts, for savages commit suicide, on occasions, when influenced by the fear of starvation, or through the dread of a lingering, painful death, or through pride. The higher psychical emotions are wanting in the savage; he is very near, indeed, in this respect, to his pithecoid ancestor; hence he bears the ills of life with all the equanimity of an animal in which aestheticized and idealized *psychos* are absent.

The semi-civilized Chinaman is, on occasions, prone to suicide; and, I am inclined to believe, most of the voluntary deaths occurring among the Chinese are brought about through pride. We know that, when overcome in battle, entire companies of these people will kill themselves rather than fall into the hands of their enemies. The Chinese are a proud, arrogant, and insular nation. They consider all foreigners as being barbarians and savages, and despise them as beings utterly beneath their notice; hence, when overcome by them, they deliberately slay themselves rather than suffer the ignominy of being slain by these "contemptible and despicable outsiders." The incentive may be, however, the fear of torture. Again, there is a certain standard of virtue that obtains among these people, which makes the fear of rape a powerful factor in engendering the act of suicide in the females of this race. The usages of war among Eastern nations has authorized, heretofore, the violation of all captured females; hence, large numbers of young girls and women kill themselves when they see that they are in danger of being taken by the enemy. This fact was especially noticed during the late war between Japan and China.

The factors inciting suicide in the Chinese and kindred races of people are not those which bring about self-slaughter in those races that are highly civilized; the psychical *materies morbi* are markedly different.

When we turn to the civilized races of the world, statistics show the curious facts that certain ethnic elements enter into the influences predisposing suicide; that voluntary death is largely on the increase; that it follows in the wake of civilization; and that its average is much higher in those races in which is to be found the greatest amount of culture and erudition.

A close study of suicide, as observed in European countries, demonstrates the fact that those nations which have their origin in the Indo-Germanic root-stocks are the most prone to commit voluntary death. With few exceptions, and these exceptions can be readily accounted for by reason of exceptional surroundings, the great centers of suicide, in which the number of suicides per million of inhabitants runs very high, are to be found in Germanic countries.

A glance at the accompanying table, prepared for me by Professor Weidner, of Vienna, for this paper, will at once show this—

TABLE I, SHOWING AVERAGE OF SUICIDES IN VARIOUS
STATES OF EUROPE FOR A PERIOD OF FIVE YEARS.*

| States. | Average Number of Suicides per Million Inhabitants. | | | | | General Average. |
	1882	1883	1884	1885	1886	Five Years.
Austria	125	123	126	129	127	126
Prussia	133	136	130	135	133	133
Hanover . . .	142	144	140	145	143	143
Mecklenburg .	168	165	170	173	171	169
Wurtemberg .	163	165	162	166	161	163
Saxony	313	311	316	314	317	314
Denmark . . .	260	262	261	260	263	261
Hamburg . . .	305	301	307	309	306	305
France	152	154	153	156	155	154
Spain.	20	19	21	18	22	20
Russia	32	35	31	35	36	33
England . . .	68	67	70	72	70	69
Italy	36	35	38	34	39	36

* I am inclined to believe that the averages in this table
are too low by two or three.—J. W., Jr.

Hovelacque demonstrates that the averages
of suicide are decidedly higher in Germanic
countries than elsewhere. The following table,
which I have slightly modified in order to
make it more explicit, appeared in *La Lin-
guistique*, in 1876 :

TABLE II, LINGUISTIC TABLE DEMONSTRATING THE PRE-
PONDERANCE OF SUICIDE IN GERMANIC RACES.
ADAPTED FROM HOVELACQUE.*

Languages.	Maximum Proportion.	Minimum of Suicides.	Average per Million.
People speaking the first group of the Italian languages derived from the Latin (Italians, Spaniards, Roumanians, Portuguese, Corsicans) . . .	74	13	31.6
People speaking the second group of Italian languages, with an infiltration of Celto-Germanic elements (French, Belgian, French-Swiss) . . .	260	36	130.0
People speaking Scandinavian, or the first subdivision of the Germanic branch (Danes. Swedes, Norwegians)	268	74	127.8
People speaking the languages derived from the Low German (Frisians, Flemings, Prussians, English, Germans of the North)	301	36	148.0
People speaking languages derived from the High German (Saxons, Central Germans, Bavarians, Austrians, Styrians, Corinthians, German-Swiss, etc.)	303	90	166
People speaking the Slavic idioms of the Southeastern branch (Russians, Galicians, Sloveni, Croats, Dalmatians)	98	14	40
People speaking the Slavic idioms of the Western branch (Czechts, Moravians, and Poles)	168	98	(130)

* Modified from tables used by Morselli in his work on Suicide.

The Celtic and Celto-Latinic races are remarkably free from the desire for self-slaughter. Especially is this true of the former in Ireland, where the average rate of suicide is only about fifteen per million of inhabitants, and of the latter in Spain, where the average is about twenty per million. From data gathered throughout Europe and Great Britain, which embrace a period of time extending from January 1, 1880, to December 31, 1893, I have constructed a table which shows the general averages of the four great divisions of European people. I have taken great care to confine my investigations, as far as possible, to cases of authentic suicide, and the following table is based on official records which were furnished by the proper legal officers and persons in authority:

TABLE III, SHOWING SUICIDAL AVERAGES OF THE FOUR GREAT DIVISIONS OF EUROPEAN PEOPLES.

Peoples.	Average per Million.	General Average.
GERMANIC.		
Scandinavians	130	
Germans of the North	155	
Germans of the South	170	116
Anglo-Saxon	73	
Flemings	52	
CELTS; CELTO-LATINS.		
Celts	32	48
Celto-Latins	65	
SLAVS.		
Slavs of the North	45	38
Slavs of the South	32	
URAL-ALTAIC.		
Magyars	52	46
Finns	40	

Morselli, in his work on suicide, observes that self-slaughter begins in the northern European states with a rather high average, which increases to a maximum in the middle states, and decreases thence slowly to a minimum in the southern states. A study of the tables already presented in this essay will show that this observation is true in every respect, although I did not have this in view when

compiling them. The general averages of the
first table will show that there was an increase
in the number of suicides, per million, in
nearly all of the states cited; if the data had
embraced a longer period of time, this increase
would have been shown clearly and emphatically in all of the states.

Wherever records have been kept for any
number of years, they always show an increase of suicide. In Sweden, where records
of the disease have been kept for a long time,
statistics show that there has been an increase, per million, of three or four for every
decade. In 1860 the average for the United
States was 32; in 1893 it was 55 for each
million of inhabitants; Ireland has crept up
from 10 per million in 1841 to 15 per million
in 1893. The average in England, in 1886,
was 70 (69+) per million of inhabitants; in
1893 it was 76 per million. In Switzerland, in
1872, it was 196; in 1893 it was 204. In Italy,
in 1886, it was 36; in 1893 it was 42. In Russia, in 1886, it was 33; in 1893 it was 40.

Two groups of periods of five years each, taken from records obtained throughout the United States, from Maine to Texas, and from New York to California, show that there is an increase in suicide in every section of the country. I do not propose to burden the reader's attention with heavy loads of official figures, therefore will make one group answer for all in establishing this fact. The following table was furnished me by Dr. L. J. Mitchell, of Chicago, medical assistant to the Coroner of Cook County, Ill.:

TABLE IV, SHOWING INCREASE IN SUICIDE PER MILLION INHABITANTS IN CHICAGO AND COOK COUNTY.

Years.	Male.	Female.	Total.	Per Million.
1890	173	43	216	144
1891	200	70	270	148
1892	228	66	274	150
1893 · · · . . .	282	83	365	182
1894	260	57	317	158
General average per year . . .	228.4	63.4	288.2	156.2

19

This table shows an increase of twelve per million of inhabitants in a period of five years. This large increase is undoubtedly due to the influence of the centennial year (1893), when the high average of 182, per million of inhabitants, was reached; leaving out this year, an annual increase of five or six will be observed, which is, probably, the natural ratio of increase for this section of the country. There are exceptional influences at work in Chicago, which create this high rate of increase, and these adjuvants to this increased average (per million of inhabitants) of suicide will be discussed elsewhere in this essay.

In Central Pennsylvania and Southern Ohio the average rate of increase is about the same. In Hamilton county, Ohio (Cincinnati), the number of suicides in 1894 was eighty-seven, an annual increase of 3.0 in five years per million of inhabitants, while in Central Pennsylvania the increase, per million, was 3.1.

In the Northwestern States an annual increase of four per million, for a period embraced by the last five years, can be noticed.* The general average of the annual increase for the United States during the period embraced by the last five years is 1.5, consequently there must be some factor at work which engenders the high averages in the localities just cited. That factor is, undoubtedly, the Germanic element (Danes, Swedes, Germans, etc.), which has heen injected into the populations of those sections where these high averages of increase prevail.

This preponderance of suicides of Germanic extraction can be noticed, locally, throughout the entire United States; in fact, if it were not for these peoples, I am confident that the general average for the United States would fall far below its present mark. In a population composed equally of Germans and Americans (Anglo-Saxons), the rate of suicide is eighty-five per cent German, and this rate does

* This paper appeared in the New York Medical Record, August 17, 1895; the reader will please bear this in mind when comparing data.

not vary throughout the entire United States.

Let us turn aside for a moment and discuss the question : Why does suicide preponderate among the German people? I do not propose to treat this subject, in this paper, with the fullness and detail that it really deserves, because, strictly speaking, it is a topic of itself and one that demands separate and individual discussion, therefore I will only enter into it incidentally.

The coroner of Cook county, Ill. (Chicago), in his last report, writes as follows : "The fact of the practice among the German race in a measure helps to bear out the theory advanced by some members of the medical profession, that the continued consumption of beer and ale is more conducive to low spirits than is that of whisky, especially when the fact is taken into consideration that among the Irish population of the city only ten committed suicide during the past twelve months. The Irishman, it is safe to assume, drinks whisky in the same proportion that his German brother consumes beer."

The idea, that beer-drinking is the cause of the preponderance of suicide among Germanic peoples, is one that is popularly accepted throughout the United States; it is, however, in my opinion, erroneous and based on faulty logic. The logician who deduces a cause from a sequence is standing on a precarious foundation; he bases his premises on an assumption—a weak and superficial basis in logical reasoning.

The English race (Anglo-Saxon) is a branch of the great Germanic race, and is a beer-drinking (ale, porter, half-and-half, beer, etc.) people, yet their average rate of suicide is, comparatively speaking, not at all high. Alcohol in any form is undoubtedly a factor in producing degeneration, and suicide is, emphatically, an evidence of degeneration; hence, I am inclined to believe that, if alcohol were the exciting cause, whisky-drinkers would more readily succumb to suicidal desire than beer-drinkers.

A careful analysis of pure malted liquors will show that they contain no ingredient capable of causing cerebral degeneration save alcohol. It is true that lupulin is toxic, but the quantity imbibed in pure beer is not sufficient, in my opinion, to occasion any great amount of degeneration.

The cause of this preponderance of suicide in Germanic peoples is not occasioned by any indulgence of the appetite, but has its origin in a psychical trait inherent in the race. As far back as history goes, both written and legendary, the Germanic races have shown a strange indifference to death. They are not braver than many other races, yet they do not seem to value life as highly as do the Celts and Celto-Latins. When the balance wheel of *psychos* loses its equipoise through degeneration, this indifference to death becomes a strong desire for death, and the German suicides; this, in my opinion, is the true cause of the high suicidal averages of the Germanic races.

Let us return now to the averages of increase as observed in the United States. The condensation of populations in circumscribed areas, viz., in cities and large towns, is a potent factor in building up increased averages of suicide. This we can readily observe by a study of mortuary statistics (suicide) as furnished by the coroners' reports emanating from all of the large cities and towns of the country. Thus, the average annual rate of increase, per million of inhabitants, for the state of New York is about 1.2, while the rate of increase for New York City is at least 4.0. These rates are calculated from the reports of the last ten years, and mean that every five years adds an average of four per million of inhabitants to the annual number of suicides occurring in New York City, and one per million of inhabitants to the number occurring in the state at large. In Chicago, as I have shown elsewhere, the rate of in-

crease, per period of five years, is annually 6.0
per million of inhabitants. This large increase is undoubtedly due to two factors: the
first is the phenomenal growth in population
of Chicago during the last five years; the
second is the large influx of Germanic peoples
within her borders. Lansing, Mich., with a
population of 20,000, has an average of three
suicides annually; this gives a rate of 150
suicides per million of inhabitants. The annual increase for the entire State of Michigan,
for a period of five years, is between 3.0 and
4.0; it is the same in Wisconsin and Minnesota.

These high averages are not to be observed
in any of the Eastern states, especially in
those states of the seaboard. It is true that
the general average of New York state is
rather high (98), but this is due to the influence of condensation of population in Brook-
lyn, New York City, and other large towns
of the state. The general average of the
state of Pennsylvania is 92; this comparatively high average is undoubtedly due to the

Germanic elements which enter so largely into its population. In Maine, Vermont, and New Hampshire, the general average deduced from official records is about thirty-eight per million of inhabitants. This average gradually decreases in the states forming the Atlantic seaboard, with the exception of the states of New York, Pennsylvania, Massachusetts, Rhode Island, and New Jersey, toward the south, until it reaches the low average of thirty per million of inhabitants in Georgia and Florida. In the Southern, Middle, and Western states the averages run from thirty to sixty, being higher in the Middle and Western states than in the Southern.

When we stop and consider that in the United States alone over four thousand people annually commit self-slaughter, and that every five years will see a material increase in this already large number, we stand amazed. Yet I have not exaggerated the estimate in the slightest degree. If I were to write down the total sum of all the people who annually make away with themselves, blank amazement, and perhaps absolute incredulity, would fill the minds of nine-tenths of those who read this article.

To those who are at all curious, this problem — *i. e.*, the total annual number of suicides in the civilized world — is one which can be easily solved. Table III. gives the general averages for the European nations, including Great Britain; to these add the general averages for the United States (55), Mexico, Central and South America (38), and Australia (65); divide the sum of these numbers by the number of averages, and this will give, approximately, the general average, per million of inhabitants, for the entire civilized population of the world.

In the United States suicide begins at a very early age. During the past ten years, almost a thousand boys and girls below the age of sixteen years have taken their own lives. In New York alone, from 1871 to the year 1876, thirty-four boys and girls committed suicide, and five of the thirty-four were between ten and fifteen years old. The records of Phila-

delphia, barring a slight increase due to condensation of population, show the correct proportion of child suicides.

TABLE V, SHOWING GENERAL AVERAGES OF SUICIDE IN
PHILADELPHIA, PA.,—MEN, WOMEN, AND CHILDREN
—FOR A PERIOD OF TEN YEARS.*

Years.	Males.	Females.	Total.	Boys.	Girls.	Total.
1884 . . .	72	17	89	1	. .	1
1885 . . .	62	16	78	2	2	4
1886 . . .	76	14	90	1	. .	1
1887 . . .	72	16	88	1	1	2
1888 . . .	71	23	94	2	3	5
1889 . . .	87	17	104	2	1	3
1890 . . .	60	20	80	2	1	3
1891 . . .	79	29	108	5	. .	1
1892 . . .	83	19	102	3	1	4 .
1893 . .	100	18	118	. .	. .	. .
General average			95	Gen'l av. . . .		2+

*Furnished by M. V. Ball, Medical Department East-
ern State Penitentiary, Philadelphia, Pa.

In this county (Daviess county, Kentucky,)
two children have committed voluntary death
in the past fifteen years—one, a boy, by hanging; the other, a girl, by poison. When I
take into consideration the extraordinary pre-
cocity of the juvenile portion of the populations of our large cities, I wonder that the
number of child suicides is not much larger.

Age undoubtedly acts as a factor in increasing or decreasing the number of those who commit self-slaughter, certain favorable ages preponderating in all the lists of suicides in my possession. From two lists of voluntary deaths, of a thousand each, taken from two periods of five years each, viz., 1882–86 and 1889–93, and from sixteen states, I have constructed the following tables:

TABLE VI, SHOWING THE INFLUENCE OF AGE ON SUICIDE.

1882–86.	Male.	Female.
Age under 10 years	. .	1
Age under 15 years	1	2
Age between 15 and 20 years	10	140
Age between 20 and 30 years	125	260
Age between 30 and 40 years	364	97
Totals	500	500
1889–93.		
Age under 10 years	. .	. .
Age under 15 years	. .	4
Age between 15 and 20 years	8	135
Age between 20 and 30 years	130	290
Age between 30 and 40 years	362	· 71
Totals	500	500

It will be at once observed that the most
favorable age for self-slaughter in women is
between the ages of twenty and thirty years,
and that in men the favorable age is between
thirty and forty. In the next table of 1,000
suicides, 500 men and 500 women, the minimum age was twenty, and the maximum age
eighty, years.

TABLE VII, SHOWING THE INFLUENCE OF AGE ON
SUICIDE.

1890–94.	Male.	Female.
Age between 20 and 30 years	110	205
Age between 30 and 40 years	203	115
Age between 40 and 50 years	102	92
Age between 50 and 60 years	56	60
Age between 60 and 70 years	19	21
Age between 70 and 80 years	10	7
Totals	500	500

It will be observed that the same law holds
good in this table also ; the favorable age for
woman lies between twenty and thirty years,
and that for man between thirty and forty

years. There is a gradual decrease in the number of suicides in women after the age of thirty, and in men after the age of forty, years.

Certain months of the year, as well as certain hours of the day, appear to be selected more frequently by persons committing voluntary death than others. Thus, there are more suicides in the United States in the months of July, August, and September than in other months, and more people commit self-slaughter between the hours of 11 A. M. and 12 M. than at any other hour during the day. It is comparatively easy to assign a physiological reason for the preponderance of suicide during the above-mentioned months, for it is a well-established fact that the hot, sultry weather of our summers acts very deleteriously on our nervous systems. It is not so easy, however, to assign a reason for the preponderance of suicide between the hours of 11 A. M. and 12 M. That this is a fact, how-

ever, a study of the following table will clearly
demonstrate :

TABLE VIII, GIVING HOUR OF SUICIDE IN 1,986 CASES.

Hour.	Cases.	Hour.	Cases.
6 A. M.	95	6 P. M.	75
7 "	60	7 "	73
8 "	102	8 "	90
9 "	110	9 "	6S
10 "	108	10 "	65
11 "	120	11 "	50
12 NOON . . .	136	12 MIDNIGHT . .	55
1 P. M.	82	1 A. M.	51
2 "	101	2 "	49
3 "	106	3 "	46
4 "	75	4 "	75
5 "	78	5 "	86
Total	1,203	Total	783

It will be seen by this table, that the suicides committed during the day largely out-
number those committed during the night;
all of my lists declare this to be a fact.

Baly and Boudin make the extraordinary
statement that the negro evinces a great pre-
dilection for suicide. This is contrary to the
proposition advanced in the first part of this

paper, *i. e.*, that suicide is of infrequent occurrence among savages.

I am not aware of the source from which MM. Baly and Boudin derive their information, but, be it whatever it may, it is wholly at variance with the statistics in my possession. We might safely answer on general principles, even if there were no records in existence, that the statement of these gentlemen is erroneous; for we know that the negro in the United States is descended from ancestors who, two or three hundreds of years ago, were utter savages; and, since it is an accepted and well-established law that suicide follows in the wake of high civilization and coincident intellectuality, it is reasonable to assume that the pure-blooded negro has not reached that degree of psychical development, which must accrue, ere the desire for voluntary death is engendered.

The pure-blooded negro is remarkably free from those forms of insanity which make themselves evident by vagaries of the higher emotions; in point of fact, he is an individual who does not possess the high psychical development of the civilized white. Says Romanes, one of the most distinguished psychologists in the world, as well as one of the profoundest thinkers: "The psychology of uncivilized man shows, in a marked degree, a kind of *vis inertiæ* as regards to any higher development. Even so highly a developed type of mind as that of the negro —submitted, too, as it has been in millions of individual cases, to close contact with minds of the most progressive type, and enjoying, as it has in many thousands of individual cases, all the advantages of liberal education—has never, so far as I can ascertain, executed one single stroke of original work in any single department of intellectual activity."

When we turn to actual evidence, we find that these psychological reasons for the non-prevalence of suicide among negroes are corroborated in every respect. In Georgia, Alabama, Louisiana, Mississippi, North Caro-

20

lina, South Carolina, Tennessee, and Virginia, where the negro is greatly *en évidence*, the average rate of suicide for the pure-blooded negro is only one in every hundred suicides. This average, in all probability, is a little too high, but owing to the lack of detail in the vital statistics of these states, it is a conservative one, and as near the actual rate as possible under the circumstances. The half-breed negro is almost invariably a degenerate individual, having inherited all of the weak physical and psychical traits of his white ancestor; consequently, the rate of suicides for mulattoes, quadroons, and octoroons is, comparatively speaking, rather high. The pure-blooded negro, like any other savage, will commit suicide on occasions, but these occasions are rare, indeed, and are brought about by the most exceptional circumstances.

The methods by which, or through which, people in the United States commit suicide, are hanging, shooting, drowning, poisoning, producing hemorrhage, asphyxiation, jump-

ing from a height, and by casting themselves
in front of a train. The proportion in which
these methods are used throughout the United
States is shown, approximately, by the following table:

TABLE IX, SHOWING THE METHOD COMMONLY USED
TO PROCURE VOLUNTARY DEATH IN THE CITY OF
MILWAUKEE, WIS.; YEAR 1894.*

Method Used.	Cases.	Males.	Females.	Average per Million Inhabitants.
Hanging	20			
Shooting	10			
Drowning	4			
Poisoning	10	X	X	X
Cutting Arteries	2			
Cutting Throat	4			
Illuminating Gas	3			
Total	53	46	7	150

* Furnished by Henry Ott, coroner, Milwaukee county,
Wisconsin.

Suicide by inhaling illuminating gas is
greatly on the increase in the Eastern and
Middle states. Says Dr. Francis Harris, medical examiner for Suffolk county (Boston),
Mass., in a letter to me, "I should add, in re-

gard to the matter of methods, that suicide by illuminating gas is rapidly increasing in this state. The case and painlessness of the method, as well as the leaving the cause always a matter of doubt as between accident and suicide, have made this method popular."

I have asserted that suicide is most frequent in those nations or communities where erudition, coincidently, civilization, is highest. We have seen that this is a fact in the countries of the Old World; now let us see if this fact obtains in the United States.

In newly settled regions of the country, say in the Western states, erudition is below par, and civilization is rude and unconventional. In these states, the average rate of suicide, per million of inhabitants, is far below that of the much older Eastern states. For purposes of comparison, I will take the states of Colorado and Massachusetts. During the last thirteen years there have occurred in Colorado (population 300,000) 102 suicides, an annual average of 28+ per million of inhabitants. In Massa-

chusetts, where erudition is higher, probably,
than in any other state of the Union, and
where the population is not influenced to any
extent by Germanic elements, the annual rate,
per million of inhabitants, reaches the high
average of 98+. The following table brings
out this fact very patently:

TABLE X, SHOWING NUMBER OF SUICIDES IN THE
STATE OF MASSACHUSETTS FOR THE PERIOD OF
TIME EMBRACED BY THE LAST FIVE YEARS,
1889-1893.*

Year.	Estimated Population.	Male.	Female.	Total.	Per Million Inhabitants.
1889 .	2,175,153	157	42	199	Approx. 91
1890 .	2,238.943	156	40	196	" 87
1891 .	2,303,536	142	45	187	" 81
1892 ·	2,369,094	211	62	273	" 115
1893 ·	2,438,363	228	62	290	" 119
Total		894	251	1,145	Gen. av., 98+

* Furnished by Francis A. Harris, M. D., Medical Examiner, Suffolk county, Mass.

Of course condensation of population must
be considered as one of the factors in the production of this high average (98 +), yet, even
when we allow for this, we will still have an
average far above that of Colorado (28 +).

IS IT THE BEGINNING OF THE END?

When we come to examine the history of
the world we find evidence that certain nations
have, at times, reached a high state of prosperity, and have then degenerated to such a
degree that they have either passed entirely
out of existence, or have lapsed into a state
of semi-barbarity. This has generally been
brought about by conquest, but the races conquered had first become enfeebled by their
habitudes of thought and manner of living.
It is a well-established fact that luxury brings
debauchery, and that debauchery occasions
degeneration. All nations that have, heretofore, reached the zenith of their prosperity,
have been engulfed, at some time or other, in
the maelstrom of luxurious habits, and have
fallen under the lethal influence of a degeneration occasioned solely by debauchery; for
the luxury and debauchery of one class brought
increased poverty on, as well as excess in, other

classes, and poverty and excess are prominent
factors in the production of degeneration, as
we shall see further on in this paper. Says
the brilliant author of "Psychopathia Sexualis," Krafft-Ebing: "Periods of moral decadence in the life of a people are always contemporaneous with times of effeminacy, sensuality, and luxury. These conditions can
only be conceived as occurring with increased
demands upon the nervous system, which must
meet these requirements. As a result of increase of nervousness, there is increase of sensuality, and, since this leads to excesses among
the masses, it undermines the foundations of
society—the morality and purity of family life.
When this is destroyed by excesses, unfaith-
fulness, and luxury, then the destruction of
the state is inevitably compassed in material,
moral, and political ruin."

Such was the condition of the Latin race
when the fierce and hardy Vandals overran
the Roman peninsula; such was the condition
of the Assyrians when Babylon fell beneath

the onslaughts of the great Macedonian; such was the condition of the Egyptians when the northern myriads swept down upon the fertile valley of the Nile, and destroyed forever the once powerful and all-conquering kingdom of the Pharaohs; and such, too, was the condition of the French nation in 1794, when Anarchy unfurled its red banner at the head of the most gigantic social revolution the world has ever known.

At the present time, community of interests, as well as higher civilization, would utterly forbid the total subjugation of one civilized nation by another, such as occurred in the olden times; hence no nation need fear annihilation from such a source. The danger comes from another point, and consists in the almost certain uprising, at some time in the future, of degenerate individuals in open warfare and rebellion against society.

The question whether the world is growing better or worse is often debated, and can be answered affirmatively on both sides. Better, because superstition, bigotry, and dogmatism have given way, to a great extent, to the tolerance and freedom of higher civilization and purer ethics in normal, healthy man ; worse, because crime (and I mean by crime *all* anti-social acts) has greatly increased on account of the pernicious influence of degeneration.

That superstition, bigotry, and dogmatism are on the wane, and that they will, sooner or later, be entombed in that depository of obsolete savage mental habitudes—absolute and utter oblivion—a glance at the success that science has achieved in the warfare waged against it by the Church, will at once declare. (Throughout this article I use the word Church to express priests of any and every denomination, whether Jew, Gentile, or Pagan, Protestant or Catholic.) A short incursion into this subject, *i. e.*, the Church's warfare on science, is absolutely necessary. For the triumph of science over its enemies—superstition, bigotry, and dogmatism, coincidently, ignorance and illiterateness—shows that the civilized world,

at the present time, is markedly different in
some respects from the world of ancient, medieval, and even comparatively recent times;
and, in summing up, this changed condition
will be a weighty factor in making up an
answer to the question which heads this paper.

When Olympus first faded away from the
enlightened eyesight of the Greeks, and
changed into space besprinkled with stars;
when Zeus no longer held his divine court on
its mystic summit; when oracles became mute
and the fabled wonders of the "Odyssey"
either vanished, or resolved themselves into
prosaic commonplaces under the investigations of the skeptic or the accidental discoverer, the Church made a most strenuous pro-
test against the destruction of its traditions.

Many of these early seekers after truth were
even killed and their goods confiscated. The
Church issued its edict against heresy (and
any doctrine that taught a belief antagonistic
to the accepted tenets of pagan mythology and
theogony was heresy), and hurled its anathe-

mas against the heretic. Olympus, in the eyes of the Church, still existed, and Zeus, the man-god, still quaffed the sacred ambrosia in its shady groves. The Sirens still sang their en-trancing songs, while Scylla and Charybdis were ever stretching out eager arms toward unwary mariners. Gigantic one-eyed Cyclops, with Polyphemus as their leader, still patrolled the shores of Sicily, and kept their "ever-watchful eyes" turned toward the open sea.

The hardy Greek sailor landed on the Cyclo-pean island, and discovered that Polyphemus, and Arges, and Brontes, and Steropes, and all the other one-eyed monsters were nothing but sea-wrack, bowlders, and weeds. He sailed farther, past Scylla and Charybdis, and dis-covered no greater dangers than sharp rocks and whirlpools. Yet farther he sailed out into the unknown sea, and the only Siren's song he heard was the whistling of the wind through the cordage of his vessel.

In vain the Church thundered against the daring investigator. Neither fire, nor sword, nor imprisonment, nor death itself could check the march of truth. Mythology and pagan theogony had received their death-blows; superstition, bigotry, and dogmatism were elbowed aside and gave place to dawning science. The Church held that that which had been believed by pious men for untold ages must necessarily be true. Science, in the garb of philosophy, with cold, dispassionate criticism, proved that these hitherto accepted truths were arrant fallacies. The poets and writers then took up the subject, and finally the people fell into line, so superstitious, bigoted, dogmatic mythology died, intellectuality took its place, and higher civilization took a step forward.

Thomas H. Huxley writes, in his preface to "Science and Christian Tradition," as follows:

"I have never 'gone out of my way' to attack the Bible or anything else; it was the dominant ecclesiasticism of my early days, which, as I believe, without any warrant from the Bible itself, thrust the book in my way.

"I had set out on a journey, with no other purpose than that of exploring a certain province of natural knowledge ; I strayed no hair's breadth from the course which it was my right and my duty to pursue ; and yet I found that, whatever route I took, before long I came to a tall and formidable looking fence. Confident as I might be in the existence of an ancient and indefeasible right of way, before me stood the thorny barrier with its comminatory notice-board —'No THOROUGHFARE. By order. MOSES.' There seemed no way over; nor did the prospect of creeping round, as I saw some do, attract me. . . . The only alternatives were either to give up my journey — which I was not minded to do — or to break the fence down and go through it."

Huxley found that this Mosaic fence, as erected by dogmatic theologians and scholasticists, was but a flimsy structure at best, and one that was easily overthrown and destroyed.

Dogmatic theology teaches that man was

created from the dust of the earth, and that he
at once fell heir to an estate of physical and
psychical habitudes which were God-like in
character; scientific investigation, on the contrary, demonstrated the fact that man's inception begins in bathybian protoplasm and
culminates, as far as his general physical
organism is concerned, in the last link of an
evolutionary chain that reaches back and
back, through countless eons of ages, to the
very beginnings of life.

The History of Life written upon the
rocky frame-work of this gray and hoary
old world, declares that man's physical being
is but the result of the laws of evolution. He did not spring into being, like
the sea-born Venus, a creature of physical
grace, and strength, and beauty; nor did the
sacred flame of an inborn intelligence at once
illumine his countenance. For thousands of
years, the forbears of the present civilized
homo sapiens were but slightly above the
Alalus (ape-like man) of Haeckel in point of

personal pulchritude; and for thousands of years, the ancestors of the civilized man of to-day were savages, with all the psychical traits of primitive peoples.

Social ethics are as much the result of evolutionary growth as is man himself. Civilization, which is but another name for ethical culture, is the outcome of the inherited experiences of thousands of years. These experiences were the results of law, and that law can be embraced in one comprehensive word — evolution.

Now, one of the most noticeable facts in biological history is the tendency that animal structures or organisms, under certain circumstances, have toward atavism or reversion to ancestral types. Not only is this to be observed in the physical organisms of animals, but also in their psychical beings as well.

Atavism is invariably the result of degeneration, as I will endeavor to demonstrate later on in this paper.

I believe that we are rapidly hurrying toward a social cataclysm, beside which the downfall of the Roman Empire, the destruction of ancient Egyptian and Babylonian civilizations, and the bloody days of the French Revolution will sink into utter insignificance. I believe, also, and think that I can demonstrate the truthfulness of my belief, that the inciting cause of this social revolution will not be found in those citizens of the United States of Anglo-Saxon and Celtic parentage, but that it will be observed among our Slavonic, Teutonic, and Latinic citizens. But, in order to furnish a parallel (from which you may draw your own conclusions), before I enter fully into the discussion of this part of my subject, I wish to review, very briefly, certain historical epochs.

When the first conquerors of Egypt, about whom history can tell us so little, first occupied the fertile valley of the Nile, the country, in all probability, was inhabited by negroes. The conquering race drove out or enslaved the native population and founded the ancient kingdom of Egypt. This kingdom waxed strong and mighty until, at the time of Rameses the Great, more than three thousand two hundred years ago, it was the most powerful monarchy in the whole world. The mighty son of Ra, Meiamoun Ra, or Rameses, as he is most generally styled, was a warrior and a statesman. He led his victorious troops north, east, and west, conquering nations as he went, until he dominated and brought into a state of vassalage over two-thirds of the then known world.

Wealth flowed into his kingdom from all the surrounding countries, consequently, luxury, with its never-failing associate, debauchery, made its appearance, and the decadence of this mighty kingdom set in.

It is true that many Pharaohs reigned after Rameses, and that the monarchy maintained its greatness for a long period of time, but luxury had taken hold on the Egyptians at the time of their greatest prosperity and had sown the seeds of degenera-

21

tion, which flourished and grew apace, until the emasculated and effeminate people yielded up their independence to the conquerors, and passed out of existence as a nation forever.

The Roman people, under the leadership of their ancient heroes, was a nation of hardy warriors and husbandmen. That preëminent military genius, Julius Cæsar, had carefully fostered this warlike spirit in the bosoms of his compatriots, and, by a series of brilliant campaigns, had made the Roman nation the most powerful on the face of the globe. The Roman legions were not only victorious on land, extending their conquests into Iberia, farther Gaul, and still farther Brittain, but the Roman triremes also swept the Mediterranean, from the Pillars of Hercules to the shores of Syria and Egypt. Wealth poured into the country from all sides, and the people reveled in a boundless prosperity.

Luxury had already begun to enervate the hardy soldiery at the time of Cæsar's assassination, yet not enough to show the full effects of degeneration and demoralization. The empire under the first emperors steadily grew richer and more powerful, and the luxury of the rich more unlimited and licentious. At length a change can be noticed. The Roman legions, hitherto victorious over every foe, are now frequently vanquished; conquered tribes uprear the standard of revolt and refuse to pay tribute; the territorial boundaries of the empire materially shrink, and its once conquered provinces pass out of its dominion forever.

The gradual degeneration of this nation is faithfully mirrored in the character of the emperors who governed it. Nero, Caligula, Tiberius, Caracalla, and Messalina, the depraved wife of Claudius and the daughter of Domitia Lepida, herself a licentious and libidinous woman, were but accentuated types of the luxurious and debauched nobility. Not only did the nobility become victims of degeneration, but the poorer classes also lost their virility, until at last we find the stability of the nation preserved through the instrumentality of foreign mercenaries. The greatness of this once widespread empire dwindled away (the freedom of its institutions contracting along with its shrinking boundaries), until we find it lapsed into a state of barbarian despotism under the son of Aurelius; and, had it not been for outside influence, it would have eventually fallen into a state of utter and complete savagery.

Now let us turn to a recent civilization. At the time of Louis XVI., the French nation was thoroughly under the influence of degeneration consequent to a luxury and licentiousness that had had a cummulative action for several hundred years. The peasantry and the inhabitants of the faubourgs, owing to their extreme poverty, itself a powerful factor in the production of degeneration, had lapsed into a state closely akin to that of their savage ancestors. The nobility were weak and effeminate, the majority of them either sexual perverts or monsters of sensuality and lechery.

The middle class, as ever the true conservators of society, seeing this miserable state of affairs, attempted to remedy it. Not fully understanding the danger of such a procedure, they allowed the degenerate element to share in their deliberations. Their moderate and sensible counsels were quickly overruled by their savage associates, who brought about a Reign of Terror (with such psychical atavists as Marat, Danton, and Robespierre at its head), the like of which the world had never seen before, nor has ever experienced since.

I have demonstrated, in the three instances of history just cited, that degeneration has invariably followed luxury, and that a social and political cataclysm has been, invariably, the result of this degeneration. That certain classes of the Old World, and of the New World, also, are living in inordinate luxury; and that certain other classes are, even now, struggling in the very depths of poverty, is a well-known fact. That this state of affairs is rapidly increasing the percentage of degenerates, such as sexual perverts, insane individuals, and congenital criminals, is not generally known; yet it is a woeful truth.

The factors in the production of degeneration are as multitudinous as they are varied, and I can find space for only a few of them. The artificiality of many peoples' lives, wherein night is turned into day, is a prominent factor in the production of degeneration. Now, the long continued influence of artificial light exerts a very deleterious effect on the nervous system; hence it is not to be wondered at that so many men and women of society are neurasthenic. Not only are those individuals who, voluntarily and preferably, spend the greater portions of their lives in artificial light, rendered nervously irritable, but those, also, who are driven by force of circumstances to turn night into day are likewise afflicted. Several years ago, I met a distinguished editor at Waukesha, who was suffering greatly from nervous exhaustion. He told me that he was so situated that he did all of his work at night, often writing until three o'clock in the morning. I advised him to quit this and to do his editorial work during daylight. Not long after, he wrote me that he had followed my advice, and that he was a new man in point of health.

The loss of nervous vitality makes itself evident by a feeling either of exhaustion or irritability. The fashionable devotee, in order to counteract this, either stimulates the system with alcohol, or exorcises the "fidgets" by the use of sedatives, such as chloral or morphia. The baneful effects of such medication are not at once appreciable, but, if continued for any length of time, they will eventually result in a total demoralization of the nervous system. Time and again have I seen fashionable men and women, at the close of the season, veritable nervous wrecks.

What necessarily would be the effect of physical and psychical lesions like these on a child begotten by such parents? The inevitable result would be degeneration in some form or other.

Again, many men and women stand the drain
of a fashionable season on their nervous systems without attempting to recoup through
the agency of drugs, and at the end find themselves physically and psychically exhausted.
They go to the seaside or some other resort,
and, in a measure, recover their nervous vitality, only to lose it again during the next season. This continues for season after season,
the nervous system all the time becoming
weaker, until some day there is a collapse,
ending in hysteria, paresis, or some other of
the hundred forms of neurotic disorder. What
will be the effect on the progeny resulting from
the union of such individuals? Again the
answer must necessarily be—degeneration.

Artificial light is not the only cause of this
nervous irritability. The long and continued
intercourse of the sexes in the ball-room, where
the women are dressed so *décolleté* that they
excite sensuality in the men, very frequently
without the men being conscious of the fact,

must necessarily exert a deleterious effect on the nervous system.

Contact of the sexes in the dance is only pleasurable because of that contact. I am fully aware of the fact that this idea is scouted and denied by those who indulge in the waltz and kindred dances. They claim that no thought of carnality ever enters into their feelings. I know from personal experience that they are honest in this declaration, yet, from a psychical standpoint, they are woefully in error. Æstheticism and carnality are by no means as dissociate as the æsthete would have us believe. *All pleasurable emotions that have their inception in the senses are, fundamentally, of carnal origin.* The waltz is æsthetic, yet all of its pleasure is based on an emotion closely akin to sensuality. Men derive no pleasure from waltzing with one another, nor do women under like circumstances.

Nature demands in the interest of health a certain amount of exercise. The luxurious society man or woman utterly disregards this

demand of nature, consequently indigestion,
with all of its associated ills, steps in, and becomes an additional factor in the production
of nervous exhaustion. To tempt the appetite, highly seasoned foods, many of which
are deleterious and injurious, are prepared
and taken into the torpid and crippled
stomach. Finally nature rebels and the unfortunate dyspeptic is forced to go through
life on a diet of oatmeal, or, weakened by
lack of healthy sustenance, the brain gives
way, and the victim passes the remainder of
his or her life in a lunatic asylum. Children
begotten by miserable invalids like these, beyond a peradventure, must necessarily be
degenerate.

Indigestion is not the only ill that nature inflicts for any disregard of her laws.
She is a rough nurse but a safe one, consequently she forbids the rearing of her
hardiest creation, man, in hot houses, as
though he were a tender exotic. The luxurious individual pampers his body, following

the dictates of his own selfish desires and utterly disregarding the laws of nature, and before he reaches middle age, discovers that he has become an old, old man, weak in body, but still weaker in mind.

The children resulting from the union of the various neurasthenics described above are necessarily degenerate. As they grow up, they show this degeneration by engaging in all kinds of licentious debauchery, and unnatural and perverted indulgences of appetite. In nine cases out of ten, they will spend the fortunes inherited from their parents in riotous debauchery, and will eventually sink, if death does not overtake them, to the level of their fellow degenerates—those who have been brought into existence by poverty and debauchery, and who await them at the foot of the social ladder. Among such degenerate beings, the doctrines of socialism, of communism, of nihilism, and of anarchy have their origin.

Now let us turn our attention to the evi-

dences of luxury and debauchery, and the
consequent evidences of degeneration, which
obtrude themselves on all sides. The reckless
extravagance of the nobility of the Old
World is well known. Vice and licentiousness even penetrate to royal households,
and princes of the blood pose as roués and
debauchees. As I have demonstrated elsewhere, degeneration in the wealthy classes of
society generally makes itself evident by the
appearance of psycho-sexual disorders. The
horrible abominations of the English nobility,
as portrayed in the revelations of Mr. Stead,
are well known. Charcot, Segalás, Féré, and
Bouvier give clear and succinct accounts of
the vast amount of sexual perversion existing
among the French, while Krafft-Ebing informs us that the German empire is cursed by
the presence of thousands of these unfortu-
nates. When we come to examine this phase
of degeneration in our own country, we find
that it is very prevalent. This is especially
noticeable in the larger cities, though we find

examples of it scattered broadcast throughout the land.

The editor of one of our leading magazines, in a remarkable series of letters, has shown that the wealthy New Yorkers revel in a luxuriousness that is absolutely startling in its license. Thousands are expended on a single banquet, while the flower bills for a single year of some of these modern Luculli would support a family of five people for three or four years! Bacchanalian orgies that dim even those of the depraved, corrupt, and degenerate Nero are of nightly occurrence.* Drunkenness, lechery, and gambling are the sports and pastimes of these ultra rich men, and it is even whispered that milady is not much behind milord in the pursuit of forbidden pleasures.

Psycho-sexual disorders are not the only evidences of degeneration in the wealthy, by any means. Many a congenital criminal is

---

* I know from personal observation that "Seeley Dinners" are of frequent occurrence in New York, as well as in other large cities.   J. W., Jr,

born in the purple, who shows his moral imbecility in many ways. Sometimes he sinks at once to the level of a common thief, but generally his education keeps him within the pale of the law. Always, however, his sensuality is unbounded, and he will hesitate at nothing in order to gratify his desires. This unbridled license has already had its effect elsewhere. We see that it has even corrupted the guardians and conservators of the public peace. The recent investigation of the police board of New York shows a degree of corruption that is simply overwhelming, and that the same state of affairs exists in Chicago, New Orleans, St. Louis, and other large cities, I have every reason to believe.

There are yet other evidences of degeneration; witness the eroticism that is to be found in our literature. Unless a book appeals to the degenerate tastes of its readers it might just as well never have been published. This is not cynicism; it is plain, unvarnished truth — witness the suc-

cess of "Trilby," of "His Private Character," of "Is This Your Son, My Lord," of
hundreds of other works of like character.
Again, turn to the stage, and we find the same
thing. The tragedies and comedies of Shake-
spear are shelved, while immoral "society
plays" and "living pictures" hold the boards.
Salacity, with only sufficient covering to hide
downright lewdness, is everywhere apparent.
Now what is the result of this? There can
be but one answer, and that is, degeneration.
That which happened centuries ago will happen again, for man is governed by the same
laws of nature now as he was then.

Statistics show that insanity is markedly on
the increase. This is not to be wondered at
when we take into consideration the fact that
debauchery is the rule, and not the exception,
among certain classes of people. Syphilis,
one of the most productive causes of degeneration, is exceedingly active throughout the
whole civilized world. Blashko states that
one out of every ten men in the city of Berlin

is tainted with this terrible malady.   This
is wholly attributable to the unbounded sensuality of the people.   Crime of every description is rearing its hydra-head, and clasp-
ing in its destroying embrace an alarming proportion of human beings.

I have shown elsewhere, that the congenital
criminal is the result of degeneration, and that
he comes from all classes of society.   He is,
however, most frequently the product of the
lower class, and lives and dies among his congeners.   I have shown, also, that the anarchist,
the nihilist, and the socialist belong to the
same category of degenerate beings.   Poverty,
brought on by high taxation, by war, and by
overcrowding, has, during the last millenary
period, been very fertile in the production of
degenerates in the Old World.   Lack of food
and sanitation, the usual adjuncts of poverty,
are powerful factors in the production of degenerate individuals.   The Old World has
gotten rid of these people as rapidly as possible by unloading them on our shores.   Year

after year, practically without restriction, thousands of these anti-social men and women have swarmed into our country, until we, comparatively speaking, a nation just born, contain as many of these undesirable citizens as any of the older nations. They still continue to enter our gates, and we ourselves are adding to their number, as I have shown, by our own production.

Some day — and I greatly fear that day is not very far distant — some professional anarchist (for there are professional anarchists as well as professional thieves) will consider the time ripe for rebellion, and, raising the fraudulent cry of "Labor against Capital!" instead of his legitimate cry of "Rapine! Murder! Booty!" will lead this army of degenerates, composed of anarchists, nihilists, sexual perverts, and congenital criminals, against society. And who will bear the brunt of this savage irruption? The ultra-rich? By no means! The great "middle class"—the true conservators of society and

22

civilization—will fight this battle. It will be
a fight between civilization and degeneration,
and civilization will carry the day. There
would have been no French revolution had
the middle class been as wise then as it is to-
day. It was taken by surprise at that savage,
bloody time, but as soon as it recovered, how
quickly it brought order out of chaos.

Education is the bulwark of civilization, and
the great middle class, freed of dogmatism, bigotry, and superstition, is welcoming education
with outstretched hands. It is gaining re-
cruits, and is strengthening its defenses, so
that when the time comes its enemies may
find it fully prepared.

From the signs of the times and the
evidence before me, I have no hesitation
in declaring that I believe that the beginning of the end is at hand! This social
cataclysm may not occur for many years, yet
the agencies through which it will finally be
evolved are even now at work, and are bring-
ing the culmination of their labors ever nearer
and nearer as time passes!

The Psychical Correlation of Religious Emotion and Sexual Desire,

BY

JAMES WEIR, Jr., M. D.

Second Edition, Greatly Enlarged and Elaborated,
Cloth, $2.00.

JOHN CLARK RIDPATH, editor Arena, says: "I have a rising belief in its truth."

THEODORE HARRIS, President Louisville Banking Company, says: "It is a long time since I read anything that gave me so much pleasure."

L. HARRISON METTLER, A. M., M. D., LL. D., says: "The argument is well taken and certainly throws much light on an obscure psychical phenomenon. I do not know that I have ever seen the question of religio-sexual correlation so clearly, so convincingly expressed."

R. T. DURRETT, President Filson (Historical) Club, says: "Whether there is any more intimate relation between the sexual and religious desires than between the desire of pleasure from seeing, hearing, feeling, etc., I know not, but there is certainly existing the correlation of which Dr. Weir speaks."

WM. ROMAINE NEWBOLD, Dean of the Department of Physiology, University of Pennsylvania, says: "That this is true (that religious emotion and sexual desire bear a double relation) there is no question."

A. M. CARTLEDGE, Professor of Surgery, Louisville Medical College, says: "Like most views Dr. Weir holds on this and kindred subjects, I fully indorse his position."

GERARD FOWKE, formerly assistant to the Superintendent of the U. S. Bureau of Ethnology, says: "The association of religion and the sexual impulse has been an enigma similar to that of the 'toughness' of ministers' sons. Galton has explained the one, and Weir has given the key to the other."

DENVER MEDICAL TIMES, July, 1897, says: "The author of this monogragh, a well known medical and scientific writer, discusses the subject from a physio-psychical standpoint. He shows the former widespread existence of phallic worship and the close relationship and interchangeableness of *libido* and religious enthusiasm. It is the first contribution of any length to the literature of this special subject, and is withal very interesting."

APPLETON'S POPULAR SCIENCE MONTHLY, Nov.,1897, says: "The author shows the connection between eroto-mania and religious mania by facts drawn from Greek and Roman history, the history of celibate religious orders, and various anthropological investigations."

————

There was only a limited number of copies of this work published in the second edition, and since it is not handled by the trade, persons desiring it should send in their orders at once. Sent on receipt of price, $2.00.

Address, Z. T. LORREY,

P. O. Box 104, Owensboro, Ky.

————

IN PREPARATION,

Psychical Traits in the Lower Animals, with Special Reference to Insects.

BY JAMES WEIR, Jr., M. D.